CLEAN
&LEAN
WARRIOR

YOUR BLUEPRINT
FOR A STRONG,
LEAN BODY

James Duigan, world-renowned wellness guru and
owner of Bodyism, London's premier health and
wellness facility, is one of the world's top personal
trainers. Bodyism's glittering client list includes
Elle Macpherson, Rosie Huntington-Whiteley,
David Gandy, Holly Valance and Hugh Grant.

KYLE BOOKS

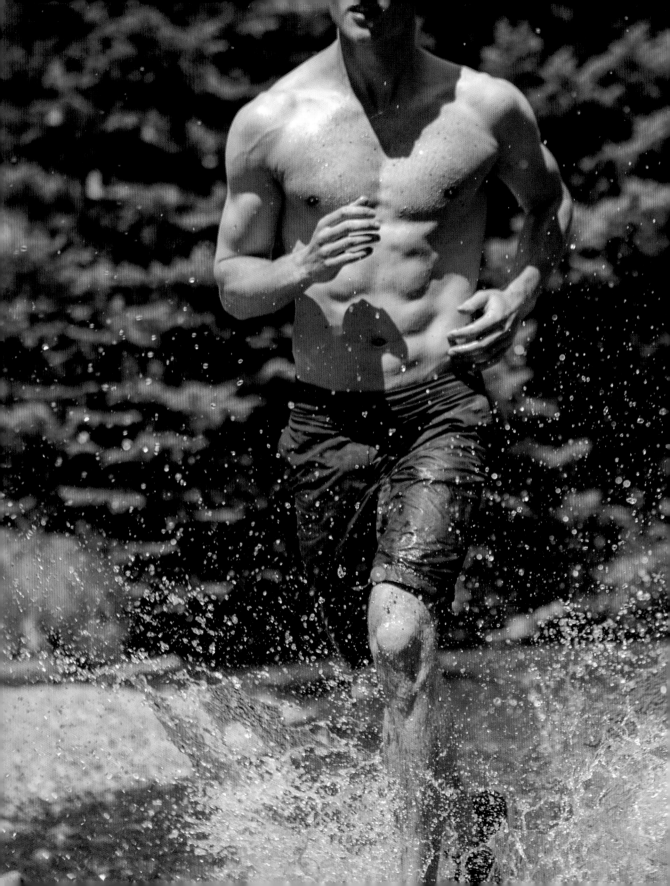

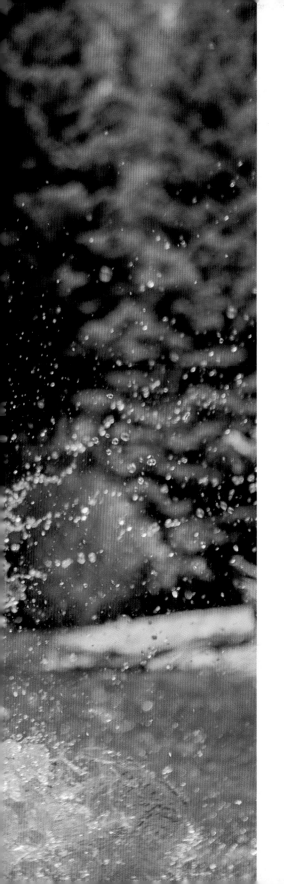

CLEAN
&LEAN
WARRIOR

YOUR BLUEPRINT FOR A STRONG, LEAN BODY

JAMES DUIGAN
with Maria Lally

PHOTOGRAPHY BY
SEBASTIAN ROOS AND
CHARLIE RICHARDS

KYLE BOOKS

First published in Great Britain in 2013 by
Kyle Books, an imprint of Kyle Cathie Ltd
23 Howland Street
London W1T 4AY
general.enquiries@kylebooks.com
www.kylebooks.com

10 9 8 7 6 5 4 3 2 1

ISBN 978 0 85783 086 9

Project Editor: Judith Hannam
Copy Editor: Anne Newman
Designer: Dale Walker
Model: Tom Puntis
Recipe Home Economy: Mima Sinclair
Recipe Styling: Olivia Wardle
Production: Nic Jones, Gemma John and Lisa Pinnell

A Cataloguing in Publication record for this title is
available from the British Library.

Colour reproduction by ALTA, London
Printed and bound in Singapore by Tien-Wah Press

The information and advice contained in this book are
intended as a general guide. Neither the author nor the
publishers can be held responsible for claims arising from
the inappropriate use of any remedy or exercise regime.
Do not attempt self-diagnosis or self-treatment for serious
or long-term conditions before consulting a medical
professional or qualified practitioner. Do not begin any
exercise programme or undertake any self-treatment while
taking other prescribed drugs or receiving therapy without
first seeking professional guidance. Always seek medical
advice if any symptoms persist.

CONTENTS

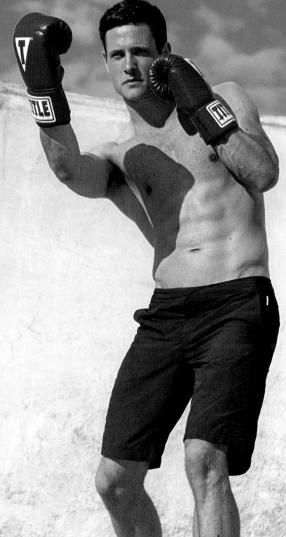

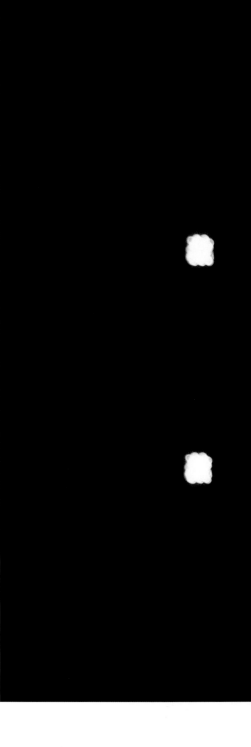

{Foreword}
by Roger Gracie

'A six-time world champion in Jiu-Jitsu, Roger is one of the most inspirational men I know.' James

My grandfather was the founder of Brazilian Jiu-Jitsu, my father was a champion fighter and my uncles and cousins fought too. So growing up, I learnt how to fight before I could even read! I started with my father when I was around two years old so I can't remember a time when I didn't fight.

When I was a little older I enrolled in Jiu-Jitsu classes. Unlike many children today, I didn't play video games in my room or eat junk. I just wanted to fight and get stronger and fitter, like my father and grandfather. My grandfather studied nutrition and didn't like us to eat anything that was artificial, sugary or hard to digest. He encouraged the whole Gracie family to eat the fresh fruit that's everywhere in Brazil, plus delicious herbs, teas and unprocessed, home-cooked food. As a result, we were all strong growing up.

By my teens I knew I was going to be a fighter. I was passionate about it and it was the only path I wanted to follow. When I fight, I feel complete – energised, alert, strong and able, both mentally and physically. I work with my body every day and I only give it the best food possible. If I fill my body with junk, it feels bad. If I fill it with healthy food, it looks, feels and performs brilliantly. You wouldn't fill a racing car with bad fuel, would you, so why fill your body with junk? I'm a fan of James' Clean & Lean approach to diet and health and I eat Clean & Lean myself.

I now have a three-year-old son and, like my father, I've started to teach him the basics of my sport. I imagine, like me, he'll grow up wanting to be a fighter too although as long as he's happy, that's all that matters to me. I'll teach him everything I know and I'll tell him what I'm about to tell you – you're a racing car, so treat yourself well and you'll achieve the best in life.

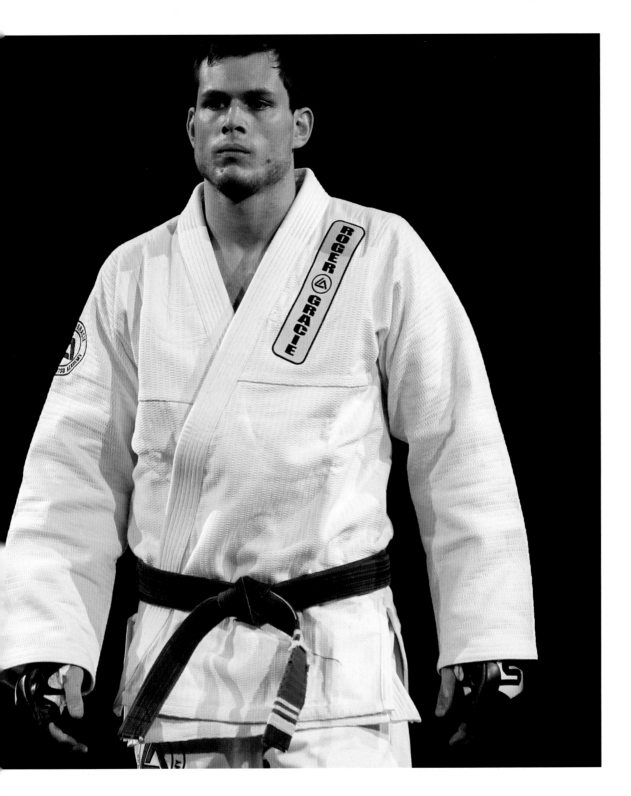

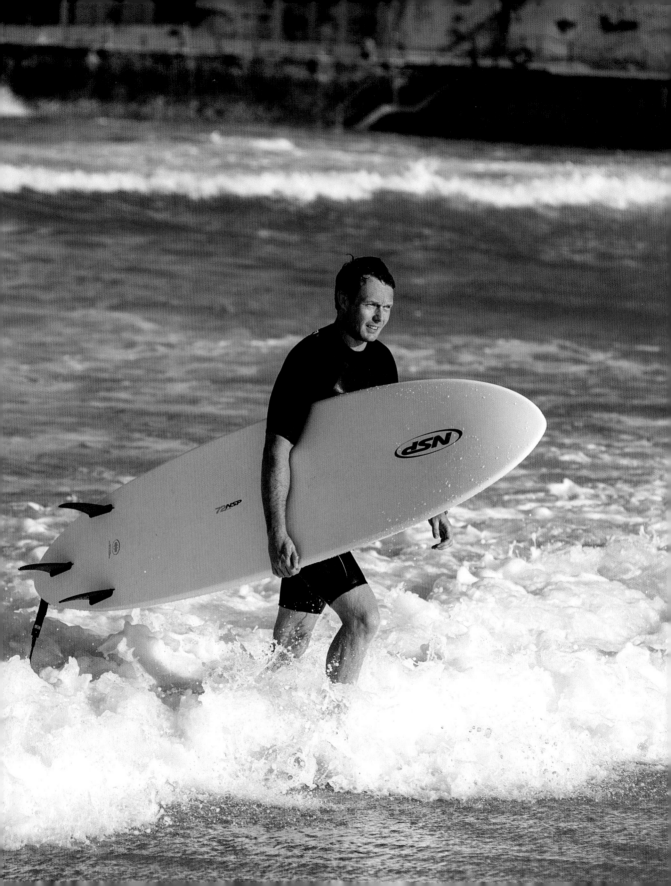

INTRODUCTION

I want you to read this book and become a better man. I want you to be physically, mentally and emotionally superior to the man you are at this very second. This is your blueprint for a strong, healthy body. I want you to feel energised, confident and happy so please don't settle for anything less.

This book is a gateway to information that will help you create a strong, lean, healthy body and will hopefully inspire you to stay Clean & Lean forever. The easy part, the part I'm really good at, is showing you exactly how to put on muscle and strip off fat, to increase your sex drive, energy and the ability to enjoy your life and to create the body you want. The tricky part is often convincing you that you deserve to feel good and yet once you understand that there is a reason for you to make better choices for yourself, it all becomes simple. So, now that we're about to get to know each other better, let me tell you this. You *do* deserve a happy life, you *do* deserve to feel good and look good. Whether we like it or not, we're all in this together and the more good, strong, honest men there are in the world, the better off we all are. I don't want to lecture you but I do want to be honest with you, really honest, so please don't be offended if I say something you disagree with. Just know that I wrote this book to help you make better decisions for your health and, by extension, for your life. My intention is to set out what I know and everything that works in a very straightforward format so that you can implement it immediately and easily. The exercise programmes have been designed with simplicity and time in mind. The food is quick, easy and delicious and every piece of information is in here to make you a better version of yourself. We have also posted up programmes and recipes on cleanandlean.com for you to buy and download when you are ready to progress beyond the book and get into more advanced territory.

Over the years I have had the privilege of meeting some of the most accomplished, successful and intelligent people in the world, from elite athletes and fighters to environmentalists, business leaders, actors, musicians and artists. All of these men have a number of things in common; qualities and habits that make them who they are. One thing that always strikes me is that you hear them say thank you – a lot. They just always seem to be grateful. They also find it easy to say sorry and mean it. They are strong enough to not have to be right about everything all the time and they also forgive those who have wronged them. This is one of the most important things you can do for your health. Any anger or resentment you hold inside is just making you sick, so forgive and move on and remember to forgive yourself for whatever you've been beating yourself up about all these years. We're all human, buddy, so give yourself a break. The other thing these guys do is look to help others, constantly. I am always amazed at how generous they are. I can tell you this much for certain since I started living my life in this way, helping others, being grateful, humble, forgiving and able to admit my mistakes, life has been amazing. I don't always get it right, I'm still learning every day and I'm definitely not perfect, but I firmly believe these are the keys to a happy, healthy life. Combine this with a commitment to excellence and what you get is a powerful human being with the ability to inspire everyone around them.

This could be you, in a heartbeat. You just need to choose it.

While writing this book, my dad got diagnosed with lung cancer. The day I found out was the scariest moment of my life. He has since completely recovered and there's a whole other book to come about that. I have also found out that I'm having a baby girl, and so I spend my time now listening to her little heartbeat in my beautiful wife's perfect tummy. Before all this happened I thought I was a pretty tough guy, but I'm not. I would often be on the floor crying about my dad, just praying for him to get better. I also cry my eyes out at every baby scan we go to. I'm not tough at all, but I'm a lot stronger than I ever imagined. Being able to tell my dad I love him and that I'm there for him, and promising my wife and baby that I will do everything I can to keep them safe and happy has given me a strength I never knew I had. It has helped me understand what it means for me to be a man. My greatest ambition in life is to be a good husband and father, to be kind, generous and gentle to my family and friends. This is what motivates me to keep going no matter what. I've given myself no choice. I've also realised that our moments of greatest adversity give us an opportunity to define who we are. How we react to these situations makes up the fabric of our lives. So choose wisely, because life is long, way too long to live not being the man you want to be. Never give up. Keep going no matter what.

Ok, thanks for listening to me. I'm grateful and honoured. And thanks for giving me the opportunity to help you. Good luck and stay strong.

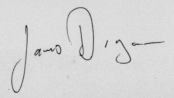

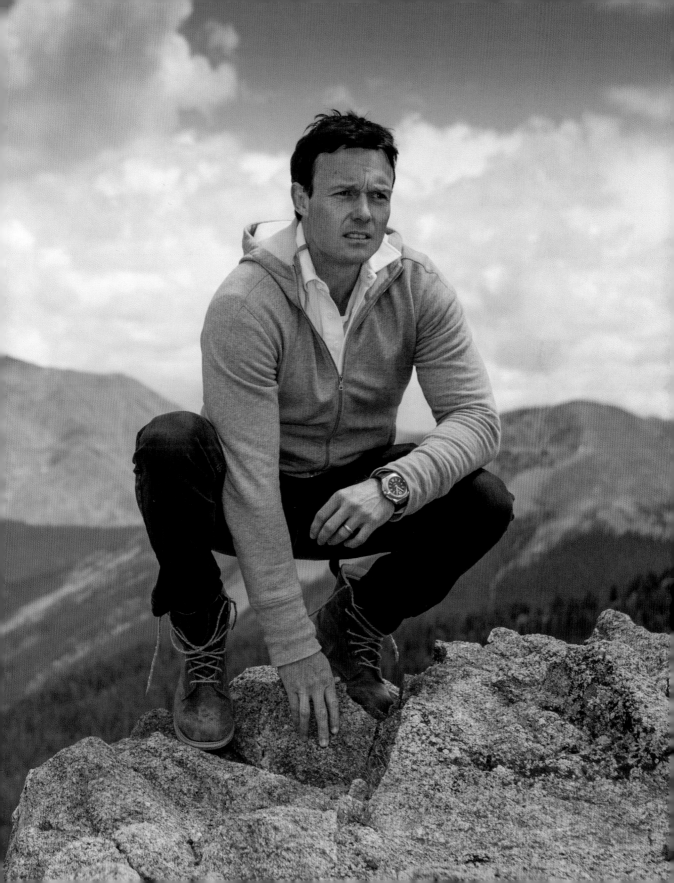

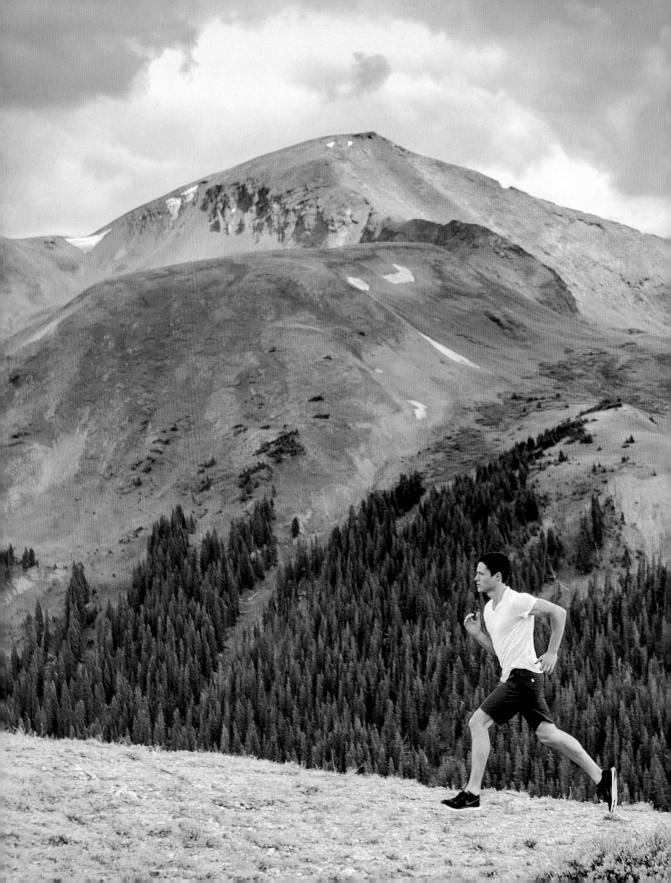

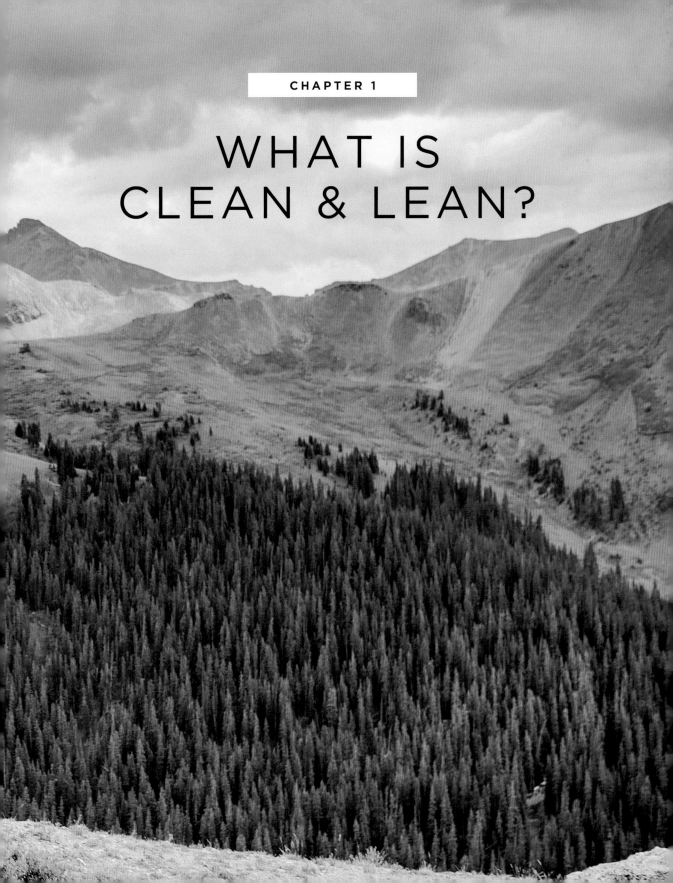

CHAPTER 1

WHAT IS CLEAN & LEAN?

Throughout the next nine chapters I'll be introducing my Clean & Lean programme. It is designed to make you stronger, faster, leaner and healthier. It has worked for hundreds of thousands of people around the world and right now I want it to work for you. All my clients are busy people who need a regime that fits around their lives, which often include working away, raising children, spending long hours in the office and a busy social life. So don't worry – I won't be asking you to spend hours in the gym or to eat meals that call for obscure ingredients and take hours to prepare. All the advice in this book is clear and easy to follow and will leave you looking and feeling strong, lean and fighting fit.

My Clean & Lean theory goes like this: a body can never be lean unless it's clean – and toxins stored in fat cells prevent this. So if you're trying to get in shape, but you're toxic, although your body will lose fat, the toxins will have nowhere to go but back into your system. You'll feel tired and weak and because your body will decide it doesn't like feeling this way, it will cling stubbornly on to fat in an effort to store the toxins more efficiently. So if you're toxic, you'll always struggle to lose weight. But if you stick to 'clean' foods, you'll lose fat quickly and develop lots of lean muscle that will help you look and feel strong and toned.

YOU CAN TELL THAT A FOOD IS 'CLEAN' IF:

✳ it has travelled from the ground, the field, the sea, the bush or the tree to your plate without a great deal happening to it along the way – for example, an apple looks pretty much the same whether it's sitting in your fruit bowl or hanging off a tree; but pasta, crisps and bread, for example, do not resemble their original state because they've been processed in a factory and 'made' into the food you see in your supermarket.

✳ it has no added salt or sugar or fake flavourings or synthetic chemicals.

✳ it doesn't last for months in your fridge or cupboard; being natural, unprocessed and toxin-free, 'clean' foods can develop mould quite quickly.

✳ it doesn't have a long list of ingredients – especially ones you can't even pronounce; in fact, a good tip is to never eat anything that contains an ingredient that you can't say (unless you have a speech impediment, in which case, ask a friend to pronounce it – if they can't then don't eat it).

✳ it doesn't list sugar as one of its first 3 ingredients.

✳ you don't feel tired, bloated or gassy after eating it.

✳ you feel energised, calm, alert and generally awesome after eating it.

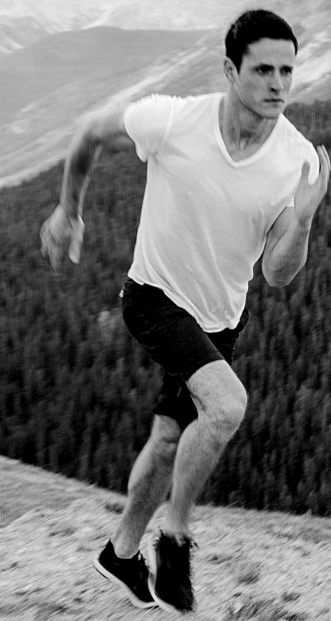

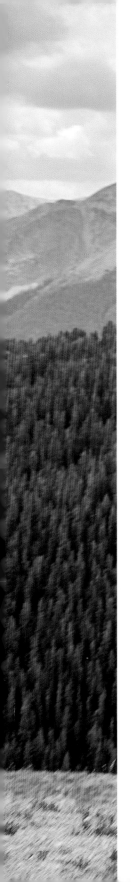

CLEAN & LEAN: THE RULES

In addition to learning to spot clean foods, there are some basic rules to follow.

1 DITCH SUGAR

In 2009, the American Heart Association (AHA) urged people to cut back on processed sugar. They said we should consume no more than six teaspoons a day, yet the average American has twenty-two teaspoons a day and many people worldwide are not far behind, while some eat even more. This staggering amount is largely made up of biscuits, sweets and fizzy drinks, plus the hidden sugar found lurking in seemingly healthy foods like cereal, bread and ready meals. To give you an idea of how much sugar we can eat in a day without realising, just one can of diet cola contains around eight teaspoons of sugar, a bowl of cereal with milk contains up to five teaspoons and a regular-sized chocolate bar contains around ten.

The first reason why you need to ditch sugar is because it makes you fat – especially around your waist and stomach. It converts to fat quicker than fat itself because it raises your insulin levels (a hormone produced by the pancreas), which leads to fat storage. Sugar is a refined carbohydrate that hits your bloodstream almost immediately, giving you a hit of energy. Your pancreas then excretes insulin to stabilise your blood-sugar levels and this causes them to drop. The result is an energy crash (hence why you often feel tired a short while after eating sugary foods). Your adrenal glands then secrete adrenaline in an attempt to boost your blood-sugar levels back up again. When your adrenal glands are overworked (I talk more about this in Chapter 4), you become even more tired. So you reach for more sugary foods to prop up your energy levels. If you regularly eat sugar, you're literally strapping yourself to an energy rollercoaster of highs and lows that will wear you out, as well as making you fat and eventually miserable. Don't fool yourself into thinking it won't happen to you. It happens all too easily.

Forty per cent of the sugar you eat is converted straight to fat (and that's if you're slim – if you're overweight, that figure can be as much as 60 per cent), and that fat is stored mainly around your stomach and waist. Sugar also stops your body from burning fat, which makes dieting and exercising even harder and more futile. Stress (and remember, sugar stresses out your system by overworking your adrenal glands) also stops your liver from burning fat. So, put simply: if you're eating sugar every day, all the gym sessions in the world won't shift the excess flab.

Sugar also robs your body of vitamins, which – as well as making it less healthy – causes it to become hungrier. A fat body can still be malnourished and that's why overweight people are always hungry: they don't eat enough vitamins to keep themselves full and satisfied. Along with mental, physical and emotional stress, sugar (which causes all these things) drains vitamin B from your body which leads to tiredness and exhaustion. If you have a stressful job, adding sugar to the mix will deplete levels of vitamin B and leave you feeling terrible. Too much sugar also lowers other vitamin and mineral stores in the body, which, over time, will weaken your immune system. Your skin will look grey, you'll struggle to get out of bed in the morning, you'll develop colds and you'll feel weak and generally below par – something you'll probably put down to your busy job or stressful life.

Sugar is also addictive. Once you start, you can't stop, because sugar has a similar effect on your brain to pain-relieving drugs (like morphine) which are known for their addictive qualities. When you eat sugar, you want more straight away – your body is craving the quick fix of energy that sugar provides. This is why it's so hard to just eat one or two biscuits out of a packet. But if you give up sugar for a few days, you lose the taste for it.

Finally, sugar wears out your internal organs because it forces them to cope with drastic changes in your body chemistry. Ultimately, it wears out your kidneys and pancreas long before their time. The sheer quantity of sugar we're all eating nowadays is also thought to be behind the increase in type 2 diabetes. This is a condition caused by too much glucose (sugar) in the blood. In a healthy person, the body is able to control blood-sugar levels with insulin. However, in people with diabetes, the body is unable to break it down properly – either because there isn't enough insulin to deal with the sugar or because the insulin isn't working properly. This is called insulin resistance. Type 1 diabetes occurs when the body doesn't produce any insulin at all, but ninety per cent of diabetes sufferers have type 2, which is often associated with being overweight, and is much more common in older people. It can be controlled through healthy eating and monitoring blood-sugar levels, but it's a progressive condition that may eventually require medication. Reduce your risk of getting it (and enduring a lifetime of monitoring and medication) by maintaining a healthy weight and avoiding sugar.

*top tip

If you think you need sugar for energy before exercise, have a banana an hour before a workout. You don't need refined sugar EVER!

SUGAR: THE WORST OFFENDERS

* **white refined sugar** (the type you get in packets and add to your coffee)
* **fruit juices:** unless your juices are freshly squeezed, you're more likely to be getting a glass of sugary water without any fibre or vitamins – the juicing process of commercial fruit juice and smoothies often heats up the fruit to the point where vitamins and goodness are lost; so squeeze your own or, better still, eat a piece of fruit (and note that the skin is where most of the goodness is, and this is often removed during the juicing process, both commercially and at home
* **white carbs,** like pasta, bread, rice and cereals; however, even seemingly healthy brown carbs (like wholemeal bread) contain sugar
* **cereal bars** are often full of sugar – they are not the healthy foods they're marketed as – and the same goes for muffins, even those called 'bran muffins' or 'breakfast muffins'; look past the marketing gimmicks and see that they're just sugary cakes made to appear healthy
* **alcohol:** it's literally all sugar

HIGH-FRUCTOSE CORN SYRUP – THE WORST TYPE OF SUGAR

High-fructose corn syrup (HFCS) should be avoided. One of the cheapest sweeteners around, HFCS encourages the release of fat-storing hormones. A study at the University of Pennsylvania in America found that it also increases the hunger hormone. It's found mainly in sweets, cereal bars, fruit drinks, ketchup, mayonnaise, some pasta sauces and even salad dressings, so always read labels and avoid it at all costs.

✻ **cakes, sweets, biscuits and ice cream** – obvious, but still worth stating

✻ **low-fat foods** – diet yogurts, most breakfast cereals, health bars, muffins and energy drinks – are all packed with sugar to give them flavour; food manufacturers often take out the fat and replace it with sugar or sweeteners, which are just as fattening

✻ **any ingredient ending in 'ose',** such as sucrose, glucose, maltose, lactose, dextrose and fructose – these are all basically sugar (another word to beware of is 'syrup')

✻ any food that lists sugar (in any form) among its first three ingredients

✻ **sweeteners** such as xylitol, sorbitol, mannitol, erythritol, aspartame, saccharin, NutraSweet, Splenda, cyclamate and sucralose; read labels and avoid foods containing any of these

HOW TO GIVE UP SUGAR

If you really love sugar, cutting it out of your diet altogether can seem daunting. But trust me, within a week you'll see a difference in the way your body looks and feels. Here's what I tell clients to do when they first go on a sugar detox:

✻ Eat plenty of chromium, which is found in eggs, liver, kidney beans, wholegrains, nuts, mushrooms and asparagus. Chromium helps control your blood-sugar levels, which, in turn, helps to banish sugar cravings.

✻ Take glutamine supplements (available in health food stores and pharmacies). Glutamine is an amino acid that reduces sugar cravings. Have one tablespoon in a small glass of water whenever you get a sugar craving.

✻ Sugar cravings are often caused by a lack of dark protein in your diet, so try eating more of this, for example, chicken legs, beef and lamb. Dark meats are high in purines which contain more satisfying nutrients than light meats like chicken breasts or fish. In fact, sugar cravings are often a result of not eating enough protein or good fat. So if you regularly have sugar cravings, increase your intake of protein and good fats (i.e. nuts, oily fish, oils and avocado) and see if it makes a difference.

✻ Body Brilliance (available at bodyism.com) is full of chromium and cinnamon, which help to regulate your blood-sugar levels. This boosts energy levels and reduces sugar cravings. I have a spoonful with water every morning and it keeps me fired up all day.

HOW TO EAT SUGAR

If you absolutely must have sugar, then there are a few rules to stick to that will go some way to limit the damage.

✻ Always eat sugar at the end of a meal. Eating your protein first (remember – you must eat some protein with every meal) leaves less room for cravings, plus it prevents blood-sugar peaks and crashes.

✻ Always go for good sugar like raw, in-season, thin-skinned fruit such as berries, grapes and apples. Or some really good-quality honey, especially manuka which contains healthy nutrients – though not too much. Once you start cutting back on sugar you'll be amazed at how quickly you lose the taste for it, and when you do have some you'll need a lot less than you did before. In fact, it will soon start to taste toxic and sickly.

✻ Never eat sugar on its own (and this includes fruit and honey). Always eat some protein and good fat with it (try a handful of nuts or a slice of meat or fish) because they slow the rate at which sugar floods into your bloodstream. If sugar hits your bloodstream too fast, you'll quickly feel high then, just as quickly, low. The slower it hits your blood, the less of a rush you'll get, which means less of a slump. If you really must have a chocolate bar, wrap it in a slice of beef with some hummus. It's amazing how quickly those sugar cravings disappear!

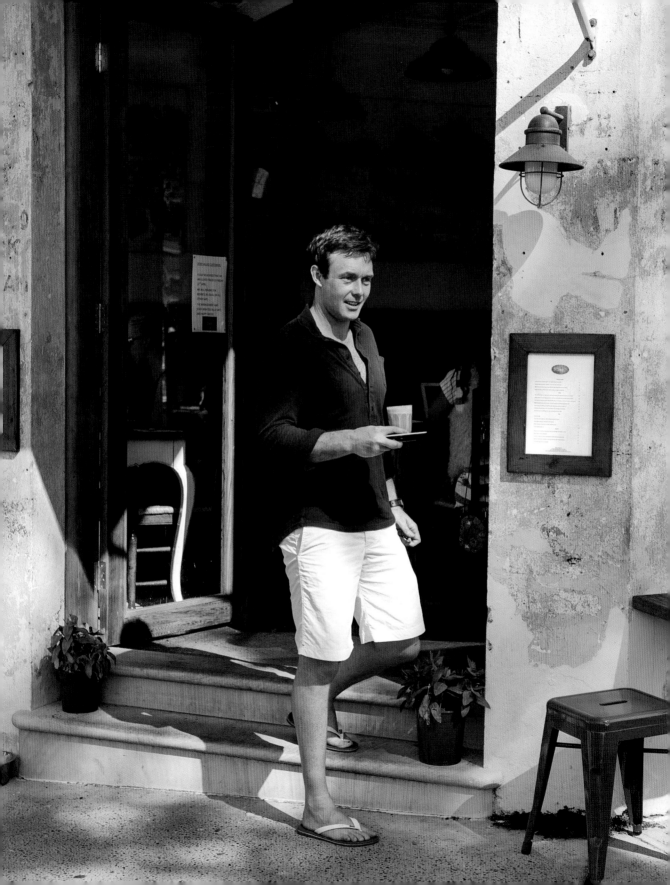

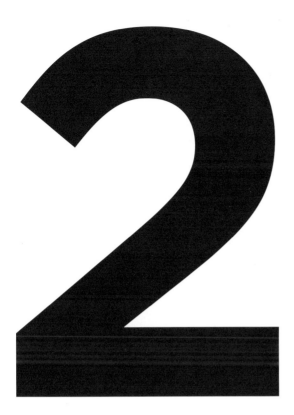

2

CUT THE CRAP*

*that's Caffeine, Refined sugar, Alcohol and Processed foods – the four main toxins that cause our bodies to cling to fat. Or CRAP.

C IS FOR CAFFEINE

This is actually fine in small doses – it can even be healthy – and I love a cup of coffee every day myself (especially just before training). One or two cups of coffee a day can help speed up your metabolism, and coffee is full of health-boosting antioxidants. Green tea also contains caffeine and you can have up to five cups of this a day (it contains less caffeine than coffee). However, most people drink far too much caffeine and it can make them fat for several reasons, which is why I've included it here. Too much caffeine can be counter-productive because it causes the stress hormone cortisol to be released as your body struggles to cope with the caffeine onslaught. Cortisol is a fat-storing hormone that encourages your body to cling to fat around your stomach and waist. People who drink too much coffee often have stressful jobs too – and, in my experience, tend to be 'stressy' types – so they get a double whammy of stress which ends up as a fat tyre around their waist.

Too much caffeine also disturbs your sleep. If you stick to one of two cups before lunchtime, you'll be fine. But if you carry on drinking coffee over lunchtime and into the afternoon – or worse, in the evening – the caffeine will affect your quality of sleep. People who claim they can drink a double espresso before bed and sleep fine are kidding themselves. They may manage to fall asleep, but they won't experience the deep, restorative sleep we all need to feel rejuvenated, and studies show that if we don't get enough of this type of sleep, our 'hunger hormones' switch on and we're more likely to crave junk food with no nutritional value. This is why we're often hungry after a bad night's sleep. If you're a new dad – and I've got tips for you in Chapter 5 – you'll know that tiredness leads to insatiable cravings for carbs. Plus the more tired you are, the more coffee you drink and, as with sugar, the cycle continues.

So if you want to be clean, lean and strong, just stick to a couple of cups of coffee a day and get your energy elsewhere (I'll show you how throughout the book, but in particular in Chapter 5). And try to avoid what I call 'junk caffeine' – the fat bombs and adult-sized big belly drinks like frappucinos and lattes with syrupy shots of flavour like vanilla. Stick to good-quality coffee with a little full-fat milk or cream and don't add sugar. If you need flavour, just add a sprinkle of cinnamon.

R IS FOR REFINED SUGAR

I've already explained why sugar makes you fat and tired (see pp. 15–17), ditch it if you want to become strong and lean.

A IS FOR ALCOHOL

This is full of sugar and, as a result, it makes you fat around the middle. It also stimulates the production of the hormone oestrogen, which further promotes fat storage around your waist and tummy. So if you're drinking a lot of beer, far from becoming more macho, you'll actually become more feminine. I see lots of new clients who drink too much beer and they tend to have rounded butts, big stomachs, man-boobs and relatively slim and feminine arms and legs. They basically look like out-of-shape women.

Alcohol is also incredibly stressful on your body, which causes more fat storage. Plus, it disrupts your blood-sugar levels and compromises your willpower – it makes you crave junk food and lowers your resistance, so you're more likely to grab a greasy burger and chips on your way home after a few drinks. Remember, too, that the liver is a fat-burning organ so when it's busy trying to process alcohol (and all the junk food it's encouraged you to eat), it stops burning fat from your regular diet. In short, too much alcohol (especially beer) will turn you into an overweight woman! So, cry me a river Man Boobs, and understand that being drunk doesn't make you more attractive, hilarious, intelligent, debonair or stylish. It's not an opportunity to test your battle skills on angry bouncers. If you are going to drink, do so in moderation and be a man about it – maintain your dignity and your trousers!

*top tip
If it didn't ever swim, fly or run – or grow off the land – don't eat it!

P IS FOR PROCESSED FOODS

These go against every Clean & Lean rule there is. Clean foods are very close to – if not the same as – their natural state. Processed foods, on the other hand, are usually made in factories, stripped of their natural goodness and pumped full of man-made additives and preservatives to make them look and taste appetising and last longer. They became really popular in the 1970s when food manufacturers realised the financial appeal of mass-producing food that lasted a long time. It's much more cost effective for them to take average- or poor-quality food and process it, adding sweeteners, colourings and preservatives, than it is to produce fresh, clean food made from good-quality ingredients that go off after a few days because nothing has been done or added to it to extend its shelf life.

An increasingly popular method of preserving processed food is to hyper heat it. But this means health-boosting vitamins, fibre and minerals are lost. That's why fresh fruit is much healthier for us than tinned fruit, which has been heated, losing much of its vitamin C along the way. Remember I said earlier that the more vitamins and minerals you get, the more nourished your body becomes? Well if you eat a lot of processed food, you won't be getting a lot of vitamins and minerals and, as a result, you'll feel tired and hungry. Scientists are also discovering more and more evidence to show that preservatives – found in nearly all processed foods – can even slow down our metabolism and interfere with our fat-burning hormones.

In general, the following are the worst processed-food offenders:

✳ Tinned foods
✳ White bread, pasta and rice
✳ Processed meats
✳ Breakfast cereals
✳ Frozen ready meals
✳ Frozen chips, wedges, etc.
✳ Packets of dried pasta
✳ Packaged cakes, biscuits, muffins
✳ Chocolate, sweets and crisps

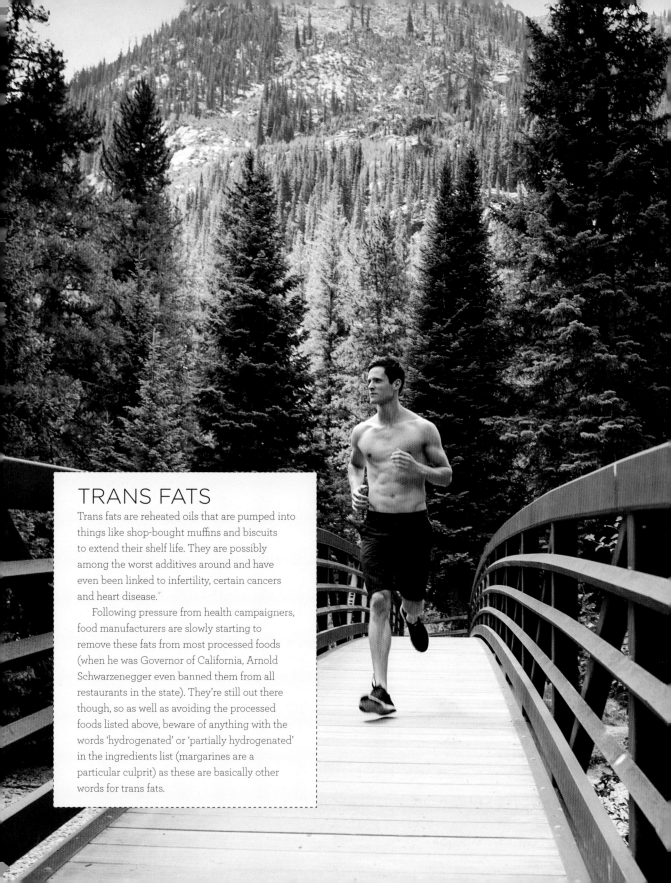

TRANS FATS

Trans fats are reheated oils that are pumped into things like shop-bought muffins and biscuits to extend their shelf life. They are possibly among the worst additives around and have even been linked to infertility, certain cancers and heart disease.

Following pressure from health campaigners, food manufacturers are slowly starting to remove these fats from most processed foods (when he was Governor of California, Arnold Schwarzenegger even banned them from all restaurants in the state). They're still out there though, so as well as avoiding the processed foods listed above, beware of anything with the words 'hydrogenated' or 'partially hydrogenated' in the ingredients list (margarines are a particular culprit) as these are basically other words for trans fats.

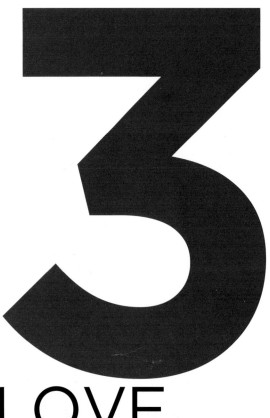

3
LOVE GOOD FAT

Don't be fat phobic and learn to love fat. When I say this, I'm talking about good fat – the heart-friendly kind found in nuts, avocados, oily fish and oils – not bad fat (the kind found on the edge of a rasher of bacon or in a pie crust). Good, clean fats should be eaten every day. They encourage your body to burn fat around your middle and to absorb vitamins and minerals more efficiently. Good fats also reduce sugar cravings, lift your energy levels and keep you feeling full for longer. They improve your concentration levels and brain power too, so if you've got a stressful job that requires you to be particularly alert and

REMINDER! WHERE ARE TOXINS FOUND?

The most fattening toxins are:

* Sugar
* Alcohol
* Fizzy drinks
* Processed foods
* Processed 'diet' foods
* Too much caffeine
* Stress

attentive, make sure you have plenty of good fats in your diet and take fish oil supplements. (See also Chapter 5, the energy chapter, for more about fat.)

THE NEXT STEP

So now you know the rules, the next step is my Clean & Lean Kickstart Plan. You can either read the rest of this book first and then begin the 14-day plan (see Chapter 6) or you can start it right now and read the other chapters as you go along.

After you've followed the 14-day plan you will feel and look amazing and be ready to stay Clean & Lean for life. I don't expect you follow every single rule all of the time. But if you try to be good 80 per cent of the time, that's a good approach. If you can manage more, better still, but don't beat yourself up if you're good just 60 per cent of the time. That's still better than nothing. I do think you'll be so blown away by the results though that you'll want to stick to my Clean & Lean regime as wholeheartedly as possible.

During the 14-day plan there will be exercises for you to do, and after that period you can try out the moves in Chapters 7 and 8 as often as you can (these are the exercises that keep male models and Hollywood actors in shape). Anything extra – a run after work, a game of basketball or a football match with your friends – is a bonus. As a general life rule, move around as much as you can. The male body is designed to lift, jump, kick and run every single day, so keep active.

Obviously, we don't have room to include all the exercise programmes in this book, so please check out www.bodyism.com for extra content and videos that you can buy and download.

MY TEN FAVOURITE FOODS BY JAMES DUIGAN

I'm going to sign off this chapter with my ten favourite foods. These are the ones I buy every week because they give me energy, feed my muscles and they taste delicious.

1. Blueberries: a superfood packed with antioxidants, which help the body deal with stress. I often have a handful with breakfast

2. Alfalfa sprouts: great in salads, soups or as a garnish – nutrient-rich, high in fibre and great for your digestion

3. Organic salmon: lots of omega fatty acids which protect the heart, plus it contains choline, which is great for improving memory and concentration. A good source of healthy fat, which can help your body burn fat – especially round the waist

4. Organic chicken: one of my favourite Clean & Lean proteins

5. Kale and asparagus: kale has powerful antioxidant properties (plus it's anti-inflammatory too) and asparagus is loaded with nutrients and antioxidants

6. Homemade hummus: eaten with raw crudités, it's the perfect snack – full of fibre, vitamins and minerals

7. Avocado: its creaminess satisfies sweet cravings, plus all the good fat and potassium can lower blood pressure. And it contains more potassium than bananas

8. Tomatoes: reduce the risk of heart disease, are high in vitamin C and are juicy and delicious

9. Chilli: adds a flavoursome punch to your food and studies have shown it can speed up your metabolism

10. Quinoa: contains all the essential amino acids for building muscles, lowers blood pressure, aids digestion and is a good source of antioxidants – so many health benefits

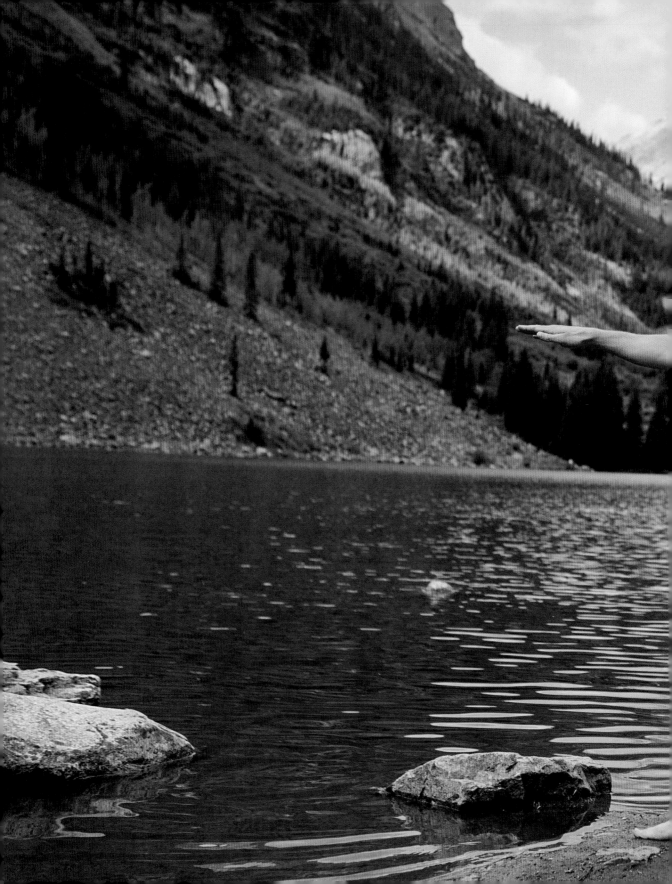

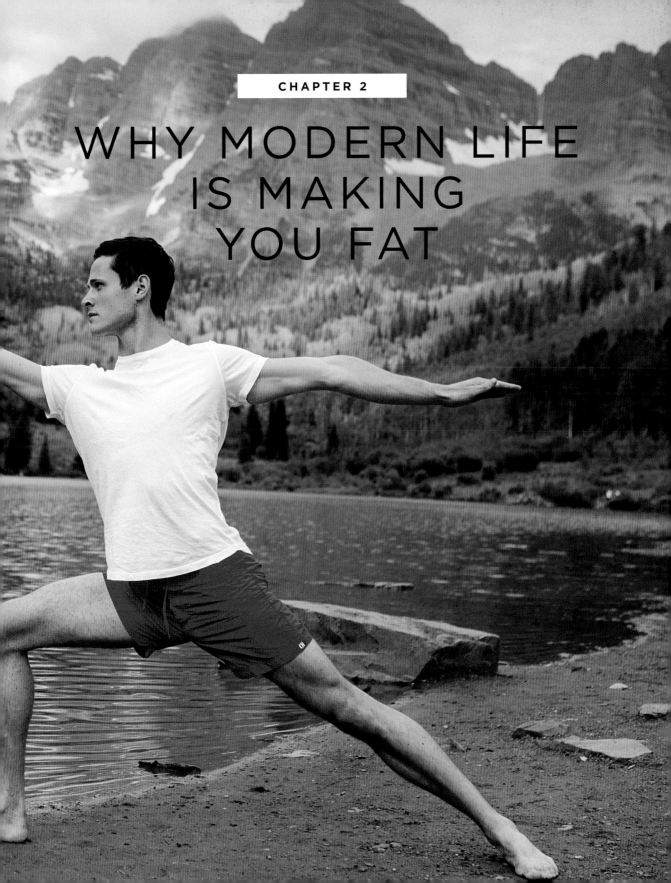

CHAPTER 2

WHY MODERN LIFE IS MAKING YOU FAT

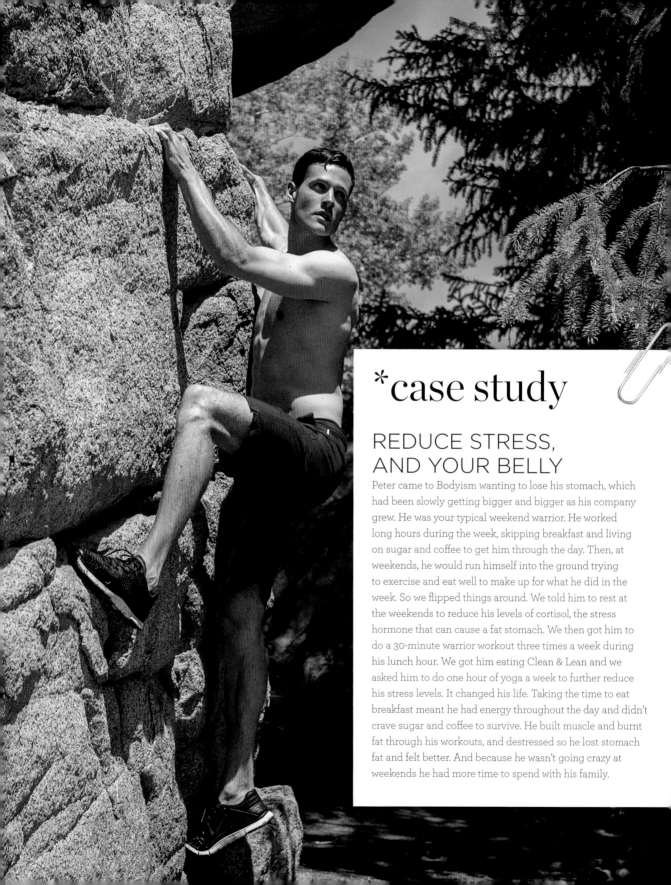

*case study

REDUCE STRESS, AND YOUR BELLY

Peter came to Bodyism wanting to lose his stomach, which had been slowly getting bigger and bigger as his company grew. He was your typical weekend warrior. He worked long hours during the week, skipping breakfast and living on sugar and coffee to get him through the day. Then, at weekends, he would run himself into the ground trying to exercise and eat well to make up for what he did in the week. So we flipped things around. We told him to rest at the weekends to reduce his levels of cortisol, the stress hormone that can cause a fat stomach. We then got him to do a 30-minute warrior workout three times a week during his lunch hour. We got him eating Clean & Lean and we asked him to do one hour of yoga a week to further reduce his stress levels. It changed his life. Taking the time to eat breakfast meant he had energy throughout the day and didn't crave sugar and coffee to survive. He built muscle and burnt fat through his workouts, and destressed so he lost stomach fat and felt better. And because he wasn't going crazy at weekends he had more time to spend with his family.

WHY YOU NEED TO FIND YOUR INNER WARRIOR

Modern man is becoming weaker and less manly. That's a pretty bold statement, but it's true. We may be making huge progress in the world of science and technology, but while our minds are becoming more brilliant, our bodies are becoming weaker and more tired. We may be living longer (thanks to amazing advances in medicine), but most men aren't living better. They're struggling to wake up in the morning and only manage it thanks to lots of coffee. Then they sit down in an office all day eating food with no nutritional value, before going home and doing the same thing there. They're not getting enough fresh air or moving around enough, which is what their body is designed to do. Instead, they're addicted to the time-killing, body-weakening habit of sitting on a sofa every night, browsing mobiles, iPads, laptops and TV screens, which stimulate their brain in such a way that sleep quality is affected and they wake up tired, looking for coffee – and the cycle continues. Is this you? If it is, then things are just about to get much better for you. Please just listen to me.

I see the results of this type of lifestyle on the streets and in my gym all the time. Men walk in for the first time beaten down by modern life, with protruding bellies, rounded shoulders, grey complexions, slim arms and legs and man boobs. This isn't how we're supposed to look and feel, guys!

Compare this image of modern man to our caveman ancestors and the warriors who lived before us. They moved around all the time, carrying heavy logs and rocks to build homes for their families. They fearlessly chased animals to eat for dinner and worked on the land all day. They protected their families. They slept well, they ate well and, as a result, their bodies were like Tarzan's – strong, lean, broad-shouldered and muscular. These guys didn't die of obesity. They probably died younger than people today due to war or a wild animal, but they would have been stronger and more energised than modern man.

They also channelled their aggression more effectively. Cavemen put the male hormone – testosterone – to good use by fighting with bears and rival cavemen or running away from danger. Modern man is still full of testosterone but often has no outlet for it, which leads to various health problems (more on that later). I'm not suggesting you start fighting with your colleagues (go play tennis with them instead), but wherever possible, you need to get back in touch with your inner warrior and channel some of that aggressive testosterone. Times may have moved on, but biology hasn't. Our bodies are still designed to move around a lot, eat wholesome, natural foods and channel aggression. That's why I'm such a huge fan of fighting exercises like jiu-jitsu and boxing for men. They blast the cobwebs off our inner warrior and leave us feeling amazing.

Throughout the rest of this book I'm going to show you how to fight, breathe, sleep and live like a warrior, but first, let's look at how to eat like one.

*top tip

It's time to man up! Take charge and change everything right now. Before you read on, get down on the floor and do ten push ups. If you can do this, I bet you already feel better. If you can't, you will really benefit from everything that is in this book. So listen up and prepare to be a warrior!

EAT LIKE A WARRIOR

When it comes to choosing what to eat or drink, rather than depriving yourself or counting calories, just make the wisest choice you can. My 'Bad, Better and Best' guides will help with this. Aim for the foods and drinks in the Best column, settle for the ones in the Better and try to avoid those in the Bad column. Although most of the foods in the Bad column live up to this name, I have shown you ways to make some of them healthier in the 'Better' column.

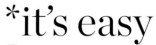

*it's easy
Green tea contains high levels of anti-oxidants and is a great alternative to coffee.

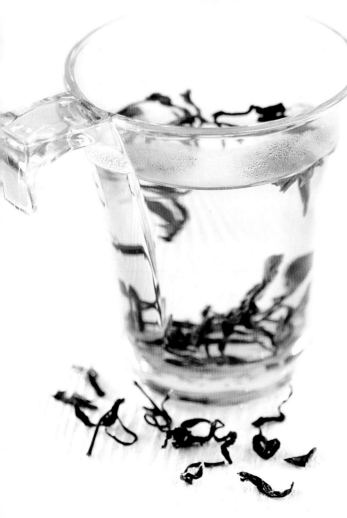

Caffeine

As I said in Chapter 1, caffeine isn't all bad, as long as you use it to your advantage. Small doses (one or two coffees, or up to five cups of green tea without sugar) will keep you alert and improve your concentration at work. They'll also speed up your metabolism and help you exercise for longer, so it's a good idea to have caffeine before a workout. Coffee, tea and green tea are also a good source of antioxidants. These are substances that protect the cells in your body from the harmful effects of free radicals found in the environment, such as pollution, tobacco smoke, UV rays from the sun and chemicals. A diet rich in antioxidants helps you feel better and wards off the ageing process.

However, just like sugar and salt, caffeine is lurking in a lot of other places. It's found in painkilling medication, chocolate and sports drinks. Caffeine is very addictive and too much raises your resistance to it, meaning you start needing more than one or two cups of coffee to keep you going. Too much caffeine also leaves you feeling jittery and unable to concentrate. It also makes you fat because it raises your stress levels, so encouraging the release of the stress hormone cortisol which makes your body cling on to fat. There's a fine line between using caffeine to your advantage and going down the slippery slope of having too much, to the point where it becomes unhealthy. So make a friend of caffeine – not a foe.

Here's my 'Bad, Better and Best' guide to drinking caffeine.

BAD	BETTER	BEST
Instant coffee – full of additives and so lacking in flavour we often add processed sugar to it just to make it taste better	Espresso	Espresso with organic cream – a small, intense amount of good-quality caffeine and the cream will help keep you full and avoid sugar cravings
Black tea – fine in theory and full of antioxidants, but you could still make it healthier . . .	Green tea – great for speeding up your metabolism and full of health-boosting antioxidants. Plus it provides a hit of caffeine to keep you alert	Caffeine-free herbal tea – peppermint tea, ginger tea, etc. (although caffeine is fine in small doses, herbal teas improve your digestion and boost energy levels)
Milk chocolate – chocolate contains caffeine, so avoid it in the evenings. Milk chocolate tends to be the most cheaply produced and is full of sugar and additives	Dark chocolate – more cocoa satisfies your chocolate craving sooner and you feel satisfied eating less	Dark chocolate with nuts – added protein slows the digestion of the sugar which prevents an energy crash. The protein will also feed your muscles
Fizzy cola (any brand) – full of sugar and fattening	Caffeine-free energy drink – fewer artificial flavours and sugar, but still not great	Fruit smoothie with nuts or seeds in it – a great hit of vitamins plus the nuts or seeds will feed your muscles and keep you full
Red Bull – raises your stress levels and is full of sugar	Guarana drink	Espresso with organic cream
Shop or café-bought iced coffee – often full of sugar	Espresso blended with ice and milk	Espresso blended with ice and organic cream
Diet pills – these nearly all contain some form of caffeine	Green tea extract	Organic green tea
Instant hot drinks – tea, coffee, hot chocolate. Processed and full of sugar	Espresso with double cream – the cream slows the effects of the caffeine	Caffeine-free/herbal tea – cutting back on caffeine reduces stress levels

Processed foods

In an ideal world I'd advise against having any processed foods. At the heart of the Clean & Lean philosophy is eating food that's 'clean' and that means unprocessed. The perfect diet consists of fresh and organic meat, fish, eggs, fruits, vegetables, nuts and seeds. In other words, the types of food our strong and lean ancestors ate. However, I'm realistic enough to know that this isn't always possible – life gets in the way (as do our taste buds) and sometimes we only have time for processed foods. Just make sure that when this happens you make your processed choices as healthy as possible.

Here's my 'Bad, Better and Best' guide to eating processed foods.

*case study

WHY YOU NEED VARIETY

Paul came to me a year ago wanting to lose his pouch on the bottom of his stomach. Paul was a creature of habit and loved his routine of waking up, eating the same breakfast, making the same lunch, then getting home and having the same dinner. Even though the majority of the foods he was eating were healthy, he was eating the same food every day. And over time, if you don't have variety in your diet, your body starts becoming resistant to those foods, even if they are healthy.

We put Paul on the 14-day Warrior Kickstart Plan and got him to have different Clean & Lean meals every day. After two weeks, Paul's pouch had flattened and he also had more energy than ever before. Paul is now no longer a creature of habit!

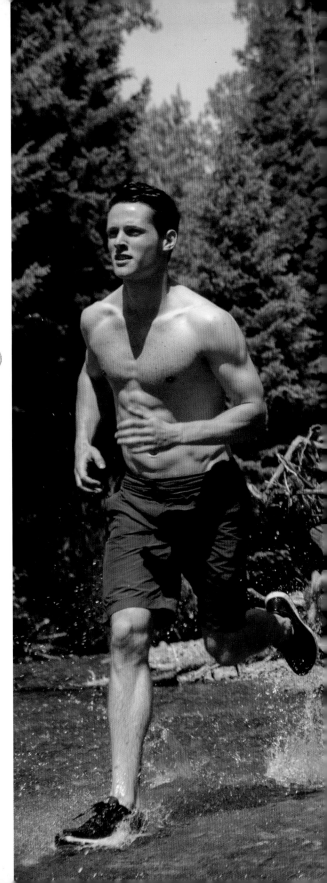

BAD	BETTER	BEST
Packaged cakes – they're full of additives and preservatives that lengthen their shelf life and artificially boost their flavour. As a result, they're full of sugar so they'll cause your blood-sugar levels to swing wildly, leaving you tired	A freshly made cake from a baker – a step in the right direction due to the fact it won't contain as many preservatives. But they're still loaded with wheat, sugar and yeast	Wheat-free, sugar-free, dairy-free muffin from a health-food store – you'll get fibre and a natural sweetener in the form of fruit
Packaged crêpes – white flour and white sugar packed with preservatives. They're a fat bomb waiting to explode, leaving you out of shape and weak	Home-made pancakes – better than shop-bought, but try and replace the white flour with either rice flour or buckwheat flour	Bodyism pancakes (see p. 126 for the recipe). Add berries or banana for extra nutrients
Ready meal with little or no protein (for example, a pasta-based dish like carbonara). This will be packed with refined white carbs, sugar, salt and bad fats and the lack of protein will leave you hungry soon after eating it	Ready meal with a decent (i.e. palm-sized or more) amount of protein (i.e. chicken or fish). This is a step in the right direction, but remember that most meat in ready meals isn't great quality, probably not organic and the meal itself will still be full of preservatives and hidden salt and sugar	A fresh ready meal with meat, vegetables and nuts or seeds that can be steamed, rather than microwaved. This won't be easy to find and it'll probably cost more than the 'Bad' or 'Better' versions, but it will leave you feeling fuller and more energised
Salami or pepperoni – the left over parts of the animal, this is heavily processed and packed with salt. It contains barely any nutrients	Slice of ham – at least you know what animal it comes from! Most pre-packaged hams are very salty though	Organic, freshly sliced lamb with hummus and avocado – a complete snack of protein, carbs and fats
Packaged salad – often dipped in chlorine to retain the colour and sprayed with preservatives to give it a long shelf life. Don't be fooled by the appearance – this food is nutritionally dead	Plastic wrapped vegetable – e.g. cucumber	Raw, unpackaged vegetables from a local greengrocer or farmers' market. This is about as fresh as it gets
Bought salad dressings – packed with sugar and salt	Balsamic vinegar and olive oil – offers a great flavour and good fats that help fill you up making it a more complete dish	Cold-pressed extra-virgin olive oil – the least processed of all oils. It's got the most nutrients and the most flavour

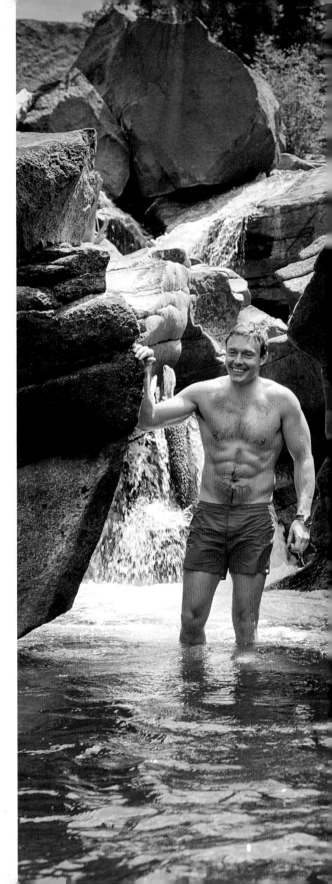

Carbohydrates

Carbohydrates are another form of sugar. However, they're ok if you work them off and have the right type of carbohydrates. If you're active and do a lot of sport, carbohydrates are vital for supplying energy, but if you sit behind a desk all day and in front of a TV all evening (or in a pub, drinking carb-heavy beer), you'll get fat. It's that simple. So don't see carbs as a bad thing – but make sure you have them as part of an active, warrior-esque life.

There's a huge difference in the quality of carbs too. White, processed ones are the worst because they can be full of sugar and preservatives and don't contain any goodness. So choose nutty, grainy, fresh brown bread over white sliced bread that has a week-long shelf life (this just shows it's full of preservatives).

Here's my 'Bad, Better and Best' guide to eating carbs.

*top tip
Don't skimp and buy cheap and low-quality foods. These usually have very little nutritional value. Invest in yourself by investing in your health. You'll feel and see the results immediately, and for life.

BAD	BETTER	BEST
White flour. Stripped of all nutrients, white flour also depletes the body of vitamin B	Wholemeal flour is a little less processed and has more fibre. However, it still contains gluten (a hard-to-digest protein)	Any gluten-free flour: corn flour, rice flour, buckwheat or millet
White bread	Brown bread	Rye bread
Wheat-based cereal	Oat-based muesli mixed with nuts	Half an avocado on a couple of wheat-free oatcakes
White pasta	Wholemeal pasta	Rice and millet, corn, vegetable or spelt pasta (gluten-free)
Cheese and ham croissant	Bagel with meat and salad	Wheat-free wrap with meat and salad (see p. 129) spelt pasta (gluten-free)
Ready-made sandwich from shop made with white bread	Rye bread sandwich	Rye bread with extra sandwich filling (tuna, chicken or meat)
A burrito	A hard-shell taco	Extra meat filling and salad – no taco
Couscous – too processed	White rice	Brown rice
Jasmine/white rice	Basmati rice	Brown/wild rice
Packaged waffles (full of sugar, salt and all kinds of other junk)	Freshly made waffles	Bodyism pancakes (see p. 126 for the recipe)
Biscuits/cookies	Rice cakes with nut butter	Rice cakes with avocado and prawns
Crisps	Kettle Chips	Salted (sea salt) celery with hummus
Peanut butter (commercial), made with salted peanuts	Unsalted peanut butter	Organic nut butter – e.g. almond, cashew and macadamia
French fries	Potato wedges	Jacket potato with some protein (prawns, hummus, etc.)
An apple Danish	A handful of dried apple	Fresh, sliced apple with almonds
Crackers	Rice cakes	Rice or oat cakes with protein (e.g. hummus)

Alcohol

Alcohol makes you fat, out of shape and exhausted. Too much beer also turns your body into a much more womanly shape because of the oestrogen levels! You can tell a heavy beer drinker by their fat, protruding stomach, relatively thin arms and legs, and rounded hips and bottom.

I don't drink alcohol at all and haven't done for years. But I appreciate that many of my clients do like a drink. The businessmen in particular often have to drink as part of their post-work socialising – either with clients or colleagues. I tell them it's OK, as long as they're eating Clean & Lean the rest of the time and as long as they don't overdo it. When you start to do the 14-day Kickstart Plan, however, I don't want you to drink at all to give your body a chance to shed toxins and stubborn fat. If you can't go fourteen days without alcohol, this isn't the book for you!

Here's my 'Bad, Better and Best' guide to drinking Clean & Lean.

WHY PROTEIN = MUSCLE

If you want to build muscle, you need protein. Exercise causes 'tears' in the fibres of your muscles and protein – found in chicken, fish, eggs, milk, yogurt, cheese, meat, legumes and chia seeds or a good-quality protein powder supplement – contains amino acids which repair and build your muscles. You should be having a portion of protein the size of your palm with every meal.

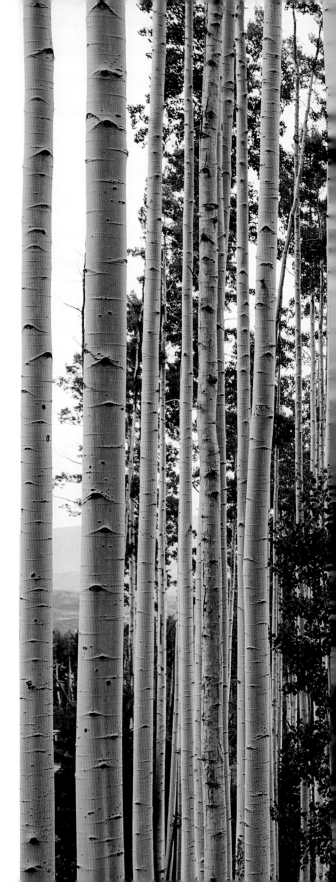

BAD	BETTER	BEST
Beer – this is packed with sugar, yeast and alcohol and is the number one fat-causing beverage in the world!	Organic beer – fewer pesticides and additives, meaning less stress on your liver (and, therefore, a cleaner system). It's still loaded with calories	Vodka, mineral water and a squeeze of lemon or lime. Grey Goose has the fewest chemicals added to it
Alcopops – packed with sugar and alcohol. Designed to taste like soft drinks, so you drink yourself fat without noticing	Vodka and juice (from concentrate) – a lot less sugar than an alcopop	Vodka and freshly squeezed juice – alcohol with some nutritional value
White wine – packed with sugar, yeast and alcohol	White wine spritzer – less sugar and less alcohol	Vodka and mineral water with fresh lemon or lime
Beer – see above	White wine – less sugar than beer	Red wine – has some antioxidants, but still a lot of sugar and alcohol
Cocktails with cola mixers – e.g. Long Island Iced Tea. Packed with sugar, fattening amounts of alcohol, plus caffeine	Cocktails with fruit mixers – fewer bad sugars and calories, so less of a fat bomb	Mocktails – non-alcoholic cocktails made with fresh juice
Vodka Red Bull – equivalent to four coffees plus a shot of alcohol. Places your internal organs under stress, ruins your sleep and all the sugar will make you fat and rot your teeth	Vodka and lemonade	Vodka and mineral water with a squeeze of lemon or lime
Shots with a milky liqueur (like Baileys) and dark spirit e.g. B52. Packed with sugar, alcohol and dairy they are a sugary fat bomb	Single shot of clear spirit – one poison instead of several. Also, less sugar	Shots are the beginning of the end! You really don't need them and your body will thank you for it in the morning if you just give them a miss
Malibu and cola – sugar with more sugar, plus caffeine and alcohol	Malibu and pineapple juice – some natural sugars, but still a fat bomb	Vodka with a fruit smoothie – clean spirit with plenty of nutrients and a little bit of fibre. Sip it slowly and enjoy the taste

Sugar

I've already talked about sugar at length (see pp. 15–17), but just to recap here – it makes you fat, tired and ages you prematurely. I always refer to it as a nuclear fat bomb exploding all over your body. Avoid it where possible.

Here's my 'Bad, Better and Best' guide to avoiding sugar.

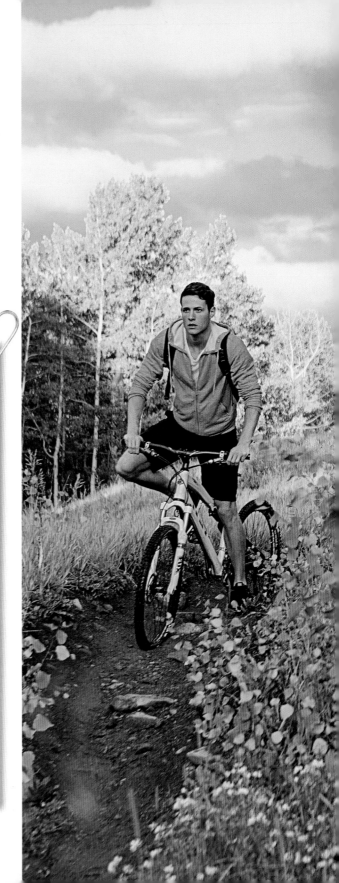

*case study

START YOUR DAY IN THE RIGHT WAY

Ralph came to us wanting to look better in a suit and to lose his belly, which had crept on over the years. He was a highly stressed, high-flying city guy who was up every morning at 5am running around Hyde Park. Then he'd eat a bowl of cereal as it was easy and quick. He thought he was doing everything right, so he couldn't understand why he was getting fat.

Ralph still trains five days a week, but we got him to sleep in for an extra hour and cut back on his running. Now he runs once in the week and again at the weekends, as well as doing the 20-minute workout three times a week during his lunch hour. Ralph now gets more sleep, which enables him to make a Clean & Lean breakfast in the morning. A longer sleep and a nutritious start to the day enables Ralph to recover from the stress at work. Since starting Clean & Lean, he has built 2kg of lean muscle, which helped him to lose his belly, and now he also looks great in a suit.

BAD	BETTER	BEST
White sugar	Brown sugar	Manuka honey
Sweets	Dried fruit	Piece of fruit
Fruit juice	Fruit smoothie	Water
Chocolate	Dark chocolate	Dark organic chocolate with nuts
Breakfast cereal	Muesli	Two poached eggs on rye toast
Dried fruit – OK as an alternative to sweets (above), but high in sugar and easy to overeat	Thick-skinned fruit salad – bananas, oranges and watermelons	Thin-skinned fruit salad – cherries, blueberries, blackberries, strawberries and raspberries. These contain more health-boosting antioxidants
Low-fat yogurt	Organic yogurt with fruit and honey	Raw organic yogurt with nuts
Ice lollies	Fruit juice	Piece of fruit
Soft drink	Fruit juice	Water
Biscuits – full of salt, sugar and bad fat	Oat cakes with nut butter	Rice cakes with turkey and avocado – the perfect blend of proteins, carbs and good fats
Ice cream – milk held together with tons of sugar. Most people can't digest dairy properly and this lowers your immune system and your ability to burn fat	Natural organic yogurt with almonds – contains a lot less sugar and the protein helps fill you up	Fresh fruit – a small handful of berries and half an apple. These are rich in antioxidants to detox your system
Muesli/granola bar – stuck together with sugar. Don't be fooled by their supposedly healthy image.	Fresh fruit and nuts – contain fruit sugars and some complete protein	Raw vegetables – broccoli, celery, carrots, cucumber and cauliflower. These are jam-packed with nutrients and have very few calories
Croissant – zero-fibre pastry soaked in bad fats. Probably the worst breakfast ever	Muffin from a health food store	Raw vegetables with organic hummus – loads of fibre, vitamins and minerals

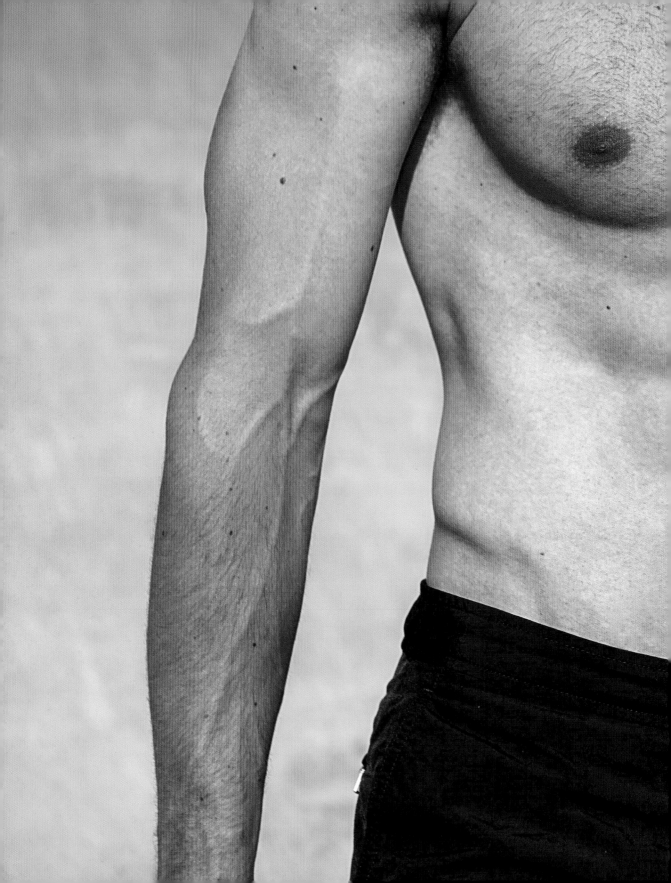

CHAPTER 3

FROM SOFT PAUNCH TO 6-PACK

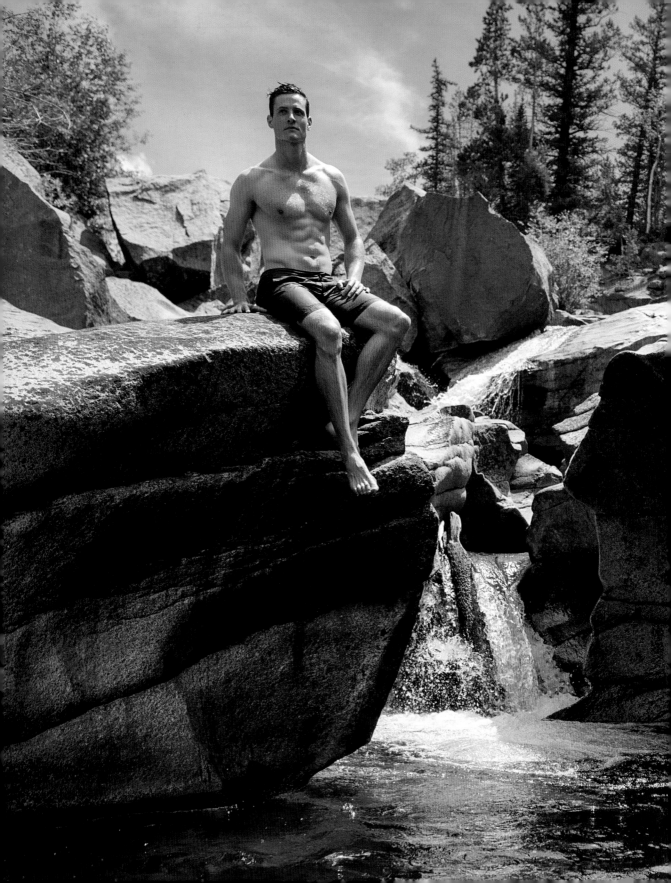

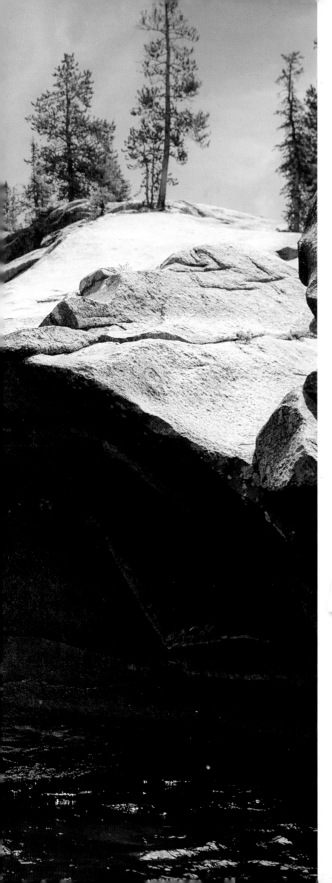

HOW TO GAIN MIDRIFF MUSCLE

Without a doubt, the stomach is the biggest area of concern for most of my male clients. I've seen all kinds of stomachs – big, hard beer bellies, swollen, distended stomachs, wobbly ones and ones that spread right around the waist and turns into back fat.

Stripping away stomach fat is fairly easy. If you eat and drink Clean & Lean, reduce stress in your life (see Chapter 4) and move like a warrior you can quickly lose your paunch and gain some midriff muscle. In Chapters 7 and 8 there are exercises that specifically target the stomach. Losing weight all over also helps you get a 6-pack – because most of us have one, it's often just a case of finding it under a layer of stomach fat.

*it's easy

If you want to step it up a gear, try the 6-day 6-pack blitz on pp. 74–81.

EAT YOUR WAY TO A FIRMER STOMACH

MY TEN FAVOURITE FOODS BY LEE MULLINS

Lee, our Director of Personal Training at Bodyism, is not only one of my dearest friends but he is one of the smartest guys in the world when it comes to nutrition and eating Clean & Lean. Here's Lee's ten favourite foods that help to make you feel amazing and stay Clean & Lean:

1. Eggs: one of the best sources of protein, plus they actually improve your good cholesterol levels

2. Sweet potatoes: full of fibre, minerals and antioxidants. They taste incredible and you stay full

3. Blueberries: loaded with disease-fighting antioxidants, as well as anti-cancer properties. They're sweet too, so they're good for snacking on

4. Avocado: a great source of oleic acid, a monounsaturated fat that has been shown to lower cholesterol. I have one most days with breakfast

5. Coconut oil: this boosts your immune system and digestion, plus it helps to burn fat. Many supermodels drink a teaspoon every morning

6. Good-quality coffee: full of antioxidants, plus it helps to burn fat when drunk before exercise. I stick to one a day though

7. Wild salmon: a great source of protein and omega-3 fatty acids for a healthy brain and heart. The protein boosts your muscles, too, and keeps you full

8. Broccoli: full of fibre and shown to help protect against prostate and skin cancers

9. Spinach: a great source of calcium and flavonoids, which contain anti-cancer properties. It's full of iron, too, which boosts your energy levels and increases muscle endurance

10. Peanut butter: opt for an organic, sugar-free type without palm oil. It tastes delicious and peanuts are a great source of antioxidants and fibre.

As well as exercising, you can also eat your way to a firmer stomach. Here are ten foods that fight stomach fat:

1. YOGURT

Studies have found that people who eat yogurt every day lose more stomach fat than those who don't. It's thought that the calcium in yogurt increases the activity of enzymes, which break down fat cells, and reduces the stress hormone cortisol, which triggers your body to store fat around your mid-section (for more on this, see Chapter 9). Keep your yogurt as Clean & Lean as possible by avoiding low-fat versions (i.e. full of sugar and sweeteners) and going for a good-quality, full-fat, Greek-style yogurt instead.

2. CHIA SEEDS

Chia seeds contain more omega-3 fatty acids than salmon, more fibre than flax seed and a wealth of antioxidants and minerals, including phosphorus, manganese, calcium, potassium and sodium. They can be eaten by mixing them into salads, yogurts or smoothies.

3. EGGS

Eggs help you build muscle because they're such a great source of protein. They also help you stay fuller for longer and several studies show that people who have eggs for breakfast tend to be slimmer and have fewer sugar cravings. Most of the nutrients are found in the yolk, including vitamin B12, which helps the body metabolise fat, so don't be tempted to have an egg-white omelette.

4. GREEN TEA

Countless studies have found that green tea helps to speed up your metabolism and increases fat burning. It contains a compound called catechin which boosts energy expenditure, increases the release of fat from fat cells (particularly around the stomach area) and speeds up the liver's ability to burn fat. It's especially effective after meals, so have a cup after your breakfast and lunch (but not dinner – it contains caffeine, so it could disrupt your sleep if you drink it too late in the day).

5. GREEN VEGETABLES

These truly deserve the name 'superfood' as they are loaded with nutrients and health benefits. Pile your plate high with as many as you like as they'll fill you up without leaving you feeling bloated.

6. BERRIES

Berries contain anthocyanins (the plant chemicals which give them their bright colour), which help to burn abdominal fat. A study from the University of Michigan in the USA found that stomach fat is more sensitive to the effects of anthocyanins than other types of body fat.

7. COCONUT OIL

The health benefits of coconut oil are phenomenal. It helps with weight loss, it can ease digestive problems such as bloating, it strengthens your immunity and it keeps your cholesterol levels healthy. You can cook with it (it's one of the few oils that retains its health benefits when heated). Pour it over just about anything, from salads to poached eggs to grilled vegetables.

8. AVOCADOS

Avocados are a rich source of monounsaturated fat, which, according to studies, helps your body work off belly fat, so always include them in your salads. Studies also show that the healthy fat in avocados helps your body absorb nutrients from salad ingredients up to five times more efficiently. Remember, a well-nourished body means more energy and fewer cravings.

9. OILY FISH

The omega-3 fatty acids in oily fish like salmon, tuna and mackerel help to burn belly fat and speed up a slow metabolism. According to one Australian study, these sources of omega-3 stabilise the glucose–insulin response of the body which leads to a fast reduction of belly fat.

10. TURKEY

This contains an amino acid called leucine, which helps prevent muscle mass loss during weight loss, plus it keeps your metabolism fired up. Like all proteins, it also keeps you full and it helps you to sleep, so include it in your evening meal a couple of times a week.

FILTER YOUR WATER

Chemicals found in tap water have been shown to mimic the female hormone oestrogen. Some studies have linked this to reduced male fertility, so always drink distilled or filtered water from a glass (not plastic) bottle.

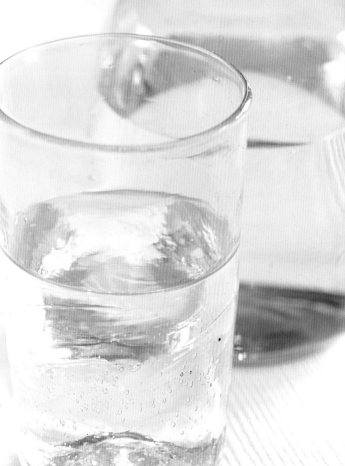

FOODS TO AVOID

Just as certain foods target stomach fat, others can cause it to be stored right where your 6-pack should be. So avoid the belly-bulgers listed below.

✳ **High-fructose corn syrup** (HFCS) is found mainly in processed foods and drinks, as I explained earlier (see p. 17), and studies show it can lead to a fatty liver and an increase in abdominal fat. According to one study at Princeton University in the USA, HFCS encourages weight gain around the waistline more than any artificial sweetener. This is because fructose is processed entirely differently in the body to other types of sugar. Read food labels carefully and avoid it at all costs.

✳ **White carbohydrates** are foods made from white flour and while they appear healthy enough – white pasta, bread and rice, for example – they're treated like sugar by your body. In other words, they convert to fat around your mid-section. Just as with sugar, refined carbohydrates can lead to extra abdominal fat if you don't burn off the quick energy they provide your body with. A study by Wake Forest University in America found refined carbs affect insulin and glucose levels, both of which are responsible for storing extra fat in the abdominal area.

✳ **Salt** can lead to water retention, which can cause excess weight in your abdominal area. Plus, added salt tends to be found in unhealthy, fatty and processed foods. Salt is also addictive – the more you have in your diet, the more you want. The worst offenders are fast food (especially chips and battered chicken/fish), salted peanuts in packets, ready meals and crisps. Having said all that, sea salt is fantastic and very healthy. It's full of vitamins and minerals and brings out the flavour of eggs, meat, fish and most foods. So bypass the cheap table salt and only buy sea salt.

✳ **Alcohol** makes you fat. We've talked about this in the previous two chapters, but I can't say it enough. It's packed with sugar and calories, which encourage fat storage around your stomach and waist. Alcohol also puts extra strain on your liver, which is responsible for metabolising fat. If your liver is processing alcohol, it's not doing the rest of its job, so your metabolism slows down which reduces your ability to burn fat. It also impacts on your willpower (meaning you're more tempted by toxic foods) and leaves you feeling hungrier and craving fatty foods the next day.

✳ **Caffeine** in drinks like tea and coffee is fine in moderation. However, studies show that too much of it causes the stress hormone cortisol to spike for eighteen hours after consumption. Cortisol (and I'll tell you more about this in Chapter 4) causes your body to cling to fat around your waist and stomach. So one or two cups of coffee a day are fine. But if you're drinking more than this, your cortisol levels will be high and you'll end up developing a little fat tyre as a result.

IS POLLUTION MAKING YOU FAT?

A recent study from Ohio State University in the US found that men exposed to dirtier air have more abdominal fat. The researchers think it's because pollutants trigger an increase in fat cells. So try to run in fresh-air areas (in a park, rather than along the side of the road, for example) and wear a cycling mask when riding on busy roads.

*top tip
Even mild dehydration stresses your body out, so it's important to drink at least 2-3 litres of still, room temperature water every single day. Sip it regularly. Filtered is best.

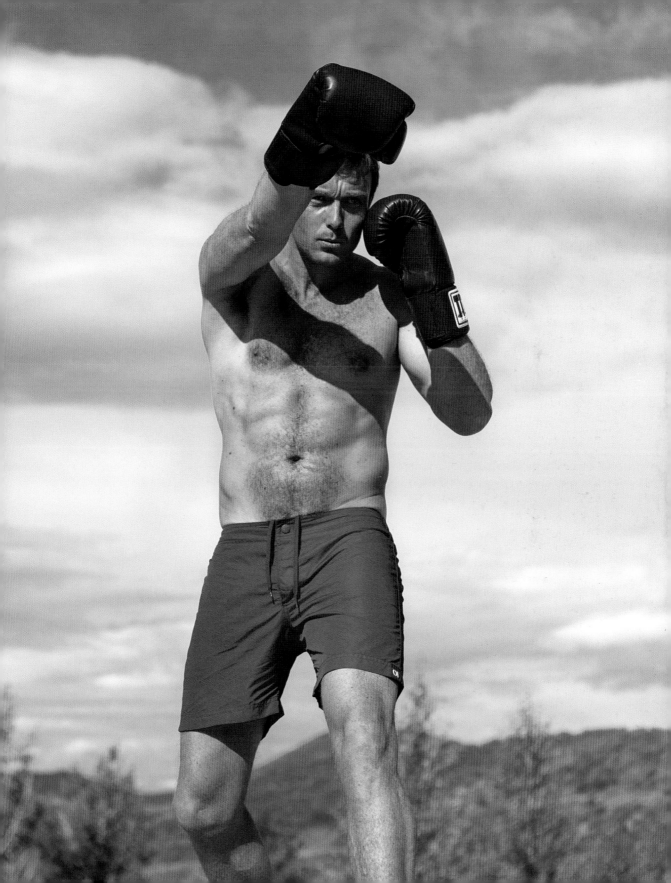

WHAT'S YOUR TUMMY TYPE?

As I said previously, I've seen all sorts of tummy types during my fifteen years as a personal trainer. As well as training Hollywood actors, athletes, fighters and male models, I also train businessmen who work eighteen-hour days and live on coffee, takeaways and stress. (Well, that's when they first come to see me, but I soon change all that.)

I've identified five different types of 'problem' stomach, each of which needs a slightly different approach to strip fat and tone up.

*it's easy

See the 14-day Warrior programme on pp. 66–73 and the 6-day 6-pack Blitz on pp. 74–81.

STOMACH TYPE 1

THE HARD BEER BELLY

This is often seen in older men who have spent years abusing their bodies. When fat is hard it means it's stuffed with toxins and this is the toughest type of fat to get rid of. A beer belly may have macho connotations, but it's basically a sign of very bad health and there's nothing even remotely ok about this. The beer belly is often accompanied by man boobs, rounded hips and bottom and spindly thin arms and legs. It's not a good look and is the result of too much alcohol, a sedentary lifestyle and making the wrong food choices over many years.

This type of stomach leads to a vicious cycle: it leaves you feeling exhausted so you can't be bothered to do anything other than sit in the pub and drink – or sit at home on your sofa – which, in turn, makes it bigger, fatter, harder and more toxic. It's also one of the most dangerous types of stomach to have and it can mean you have lots of fat wrapped around vital internal organs. This increases your risk of heart disease, type 2 diabetes and various cancers.

Flatten-it plan

Unfortunately, there's no quick fix for this type of stomach, so you need to overhaul your life and get Clean & Lean. Follow all the recommendations in this book, paying particular attention to the advice on avoiding alcohol, sugar and processed foods (see pp. 19–20).

STOMACH TYPE 2

YOU'RE FIT BUT FAT

I see very fit men who cycle to work every day and regularly run half marathons who are fit, look slim in their clothes, but have fat little stomachs. This type of belly isn't as dangerous as the beer belly (left) but it can head that way as you get older (especially if you're not following Clean & Lean). Plus, it looks terrible.

Flatten-it plan

Mix up your exercise. In most cases, this type of belly is caused by either not enough exercise or doing the same type of exercise (usually cardio) over and over again. Cardiovascular exercises like running or cycling are fine in theory – they burn fat and they're great for your heart (hence the name). But they can also put your body under stress if you constantly overdo it, which raises cortisol levels. This encourages your body to cling to fat around your stomach.

So instead of advising you to go out to do more exercise, I actually say you should do a little less and replace half of your cardio sessions with some yoga, Pilates or weight-bearing exercises (see Chapter 8 for ideas). I also recommend taking daily fish oil supplements to blitz this type of stomach fat, as well as including oily fish in your weekly diet (aim for three portions of salmon, mackerel or sardines a week).

YOU'VE GOT A FAT BACK

Lots of guys have fat that spreads across the stomach, round to the sides of their waist and creeps around their lower back. They literally have belt hang from every angle. This type of shape tends to be caused by stress and too much sugar.

Flatten-it plan

Try to reduce stress in your life, and that includes destressing your diet (see Chapter 4 for more about this). You will also benefit from some back-toning exercises, which I've included in Chapter 8. Also eliminate sugar as much as possible (he's not your friend, so stop seeing him).

SKINNY STOMACH

Some of my younger clients complain they have a skinny, androgynous stomach that's flat, but muscle-free. These guys tend not to be able to put on weight very easily and hate their shapeless look.

Bulk-it-up plan

If you have a skinny stomach you need to eat like a caveman, eating protein with every single meal and snack. You also need to do some exercises that will increase your testosterone levels, such as squats and dead lifts (see Chapter 8 for more on these). Plus you should try a fighting sport like wrestling or jiu jitsu. It increases testosterone and confidence.

LITTLE POOCH STOMACH

Some men suffer from bloating in the same way as women and, while they can be slim all over, they have a sticky-out, pooch-like stomach that won't shift. It's nearly always caused by stress and the wrong types of food. Sometimes it's caused by eating a food that doesn't work for your body. This can happen over time if you keep eating the same foods and don't get enough variety in your diet. When you eat the same foods over and over again, our bodies become less sensitive to them to the point that the food begins to act as a stress on the body. The way this often shows is a small pouch of fat around and below our belly button.

Flatten-it plan

You need to reduce your stress levels to reduce stomach fat and bloating. Go for lots of walks (this has the added benefit of improving your digestion), do stress-busting exercises like yoga and eat foods that reduce stress (see Chapter 4). Get a greater variety of Clean & Lean foods in your diet. I often tell my clients that when they go for their weekly food shop, they should add a new food they haven't tried before (or haven't eaten in a long time). As long as it is a Clean & Lean food, after eating it you should feel energised and amazing as your body will have received a hit of nutrients it may not have had in a while.

*top tip

If you want to increase your protein but can't face meat, add a scoop of our Body Brilliance (bodyism.com or cleanandlean.com) to yogurt, pancakes, smoothies, quinoa (the possibilities are endless).

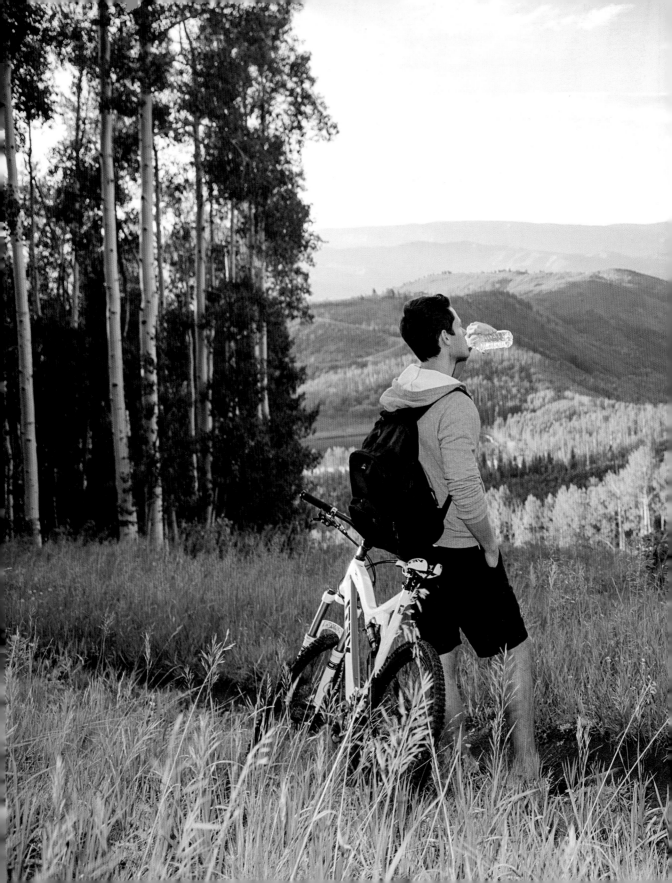

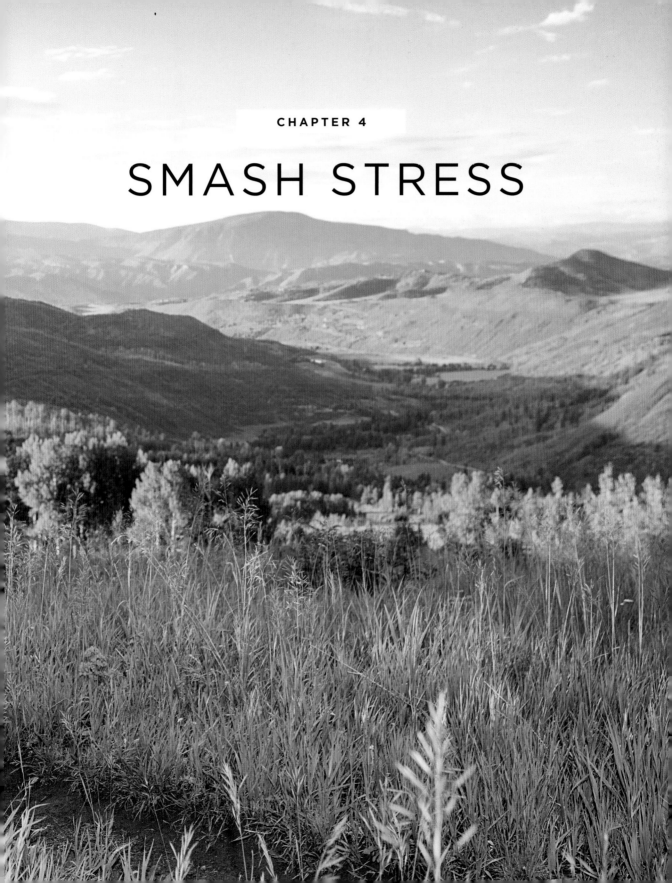

CHAPTER 4

SMASH STRESS

SMASH STRESS

A little bit of stress is great. It fires up your inner warrior and makes you work harder and strive for better things. If you never got stressed, you'd lack the motivation to get out of bed in the mornings, work hard at your job and relationships and generally live a fulfilled life.

When we feel stressed, our body releases two hormones – adrenaline and cortisol. Together, they work to power up our muscles and mind so we can take on whatever stressful situation is upon us.

Hundreds of years ago, these hormones kept our warrior ancestors out of trouble. If a tiger approached them or their family, the stress they felt gave them a shot of extra energy to run away or stay and fight. It's where the expression 'fight or flight' comes from. But modern-day stress doesn't involve tigers (if it did, we could post a picture of it on twitter). It involves endless deadlines, long hours, bosses who micromanage or bully, employees who don't pull their weight, train delays, money worries and relationship issues. But we get that same hit of adrenaline and cortisol to deal with it. So if you regularly feel stressed by life's small annoyances – and let's face it, who doesn't? – your body is being drip-fed stress hormones all day long.

Why is this a bad thing? Well, if you had to run away from, or wrestle with, a tiger you would burn off the adrenaline. But when you feel stressed by a train delay or a credit card bill, you just sit there seething while the cortisol and adrenaline flood your system. These hormones raise your heart rate (fine, if you need to run away – but not if you don't) and cause you to take shallow breaths, leaving you jittery and suffering from headaches. They also encourage your body to cling to fat and they wear out your adrenal glands (see below). Over time, if you don't handle your stress levels or find an outlet for them, you can accumulate a lot of suppressed rage which causes your body to pump out more adrenaline and cortisol, and so the cycle continues. That's why you have to find your inner warrior and fight your way out of this stress trap!

ARE YOU WEARING OUT YOUR ADRENAL GLANDS?

You adrenals are tiny triangular glands that are situated just above the kidneys and release hormones like cortisol into the system when they are stressed. These glands are only meant for emergencies – like running into a tiger – they're not designed to be overworked every single day. But we live in a 24/7 society and we're working harder than ever, exercising less and eating more junk. All day long our bodies are coming under stress and our poor overworked adrenals are pumping out cortisol as a result.

When they first come to see me, many of my clients' adrenal glands are overworked. Symptoms include a lowered immune system, tiredness, fatigue, constant colds and depression. Sleep is affected too because the body's too wired (from the cortisol and adrenaline) to wind down in the evenings. When your adrenal glands are worn out your digestive system also slows down which can often leave you constipated, bloated and toxic.

In short, modern life is zapping modern man's strength. The solution? Become a warrior! Blitz your stress and channel your rage into fighting exercises like ju-jitsu and hanging out with your friends playing your favourite sport. Lots of men do this when they're younger, but when family and work come along they feel they can't spare the time. However, it's vital that you make time for exactly this – it will reduce your stress levels and keep you fighting fit.

*top tip

Do you often feel irritable and tired and suffer from insomnia? A recent study found that a deficiency in the B vitamin folate can lead to all these things. Boost your intake of this vitamin – good sources include kidney beans, lentils, spinach and lettuce, so tuck in to plenty of these foods if you feel cranky.

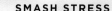
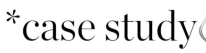

*case study

WHERE'S THE FUN IN YOUR LIFE?

A client of mine once told me a story that sums up this theory perfectly. He was in his mid-thirties and had a beautiful wife and two children. He had a high-powered job in the city and a large house just outside of London. In short, his life was 'perfect on paper'. He had ticked all the boxes he was 'supposed to' by his age. But he wasn't happy. He felt stressed and depressed a lot of the time. Because of this, he was drinking coffee all day long to keep his energy levels up and he was drinking wine every night in an attempt to wind down and, as he explained, 'soften the corners' of his negative and anxious thoughts. This toxic combination of stress, caffeine and alcohol was making him feel worse, not better. Things came to a head when he broke down on his way to work one morning. He saw his GP who directed him to therapy.

One of the first things the therapist asked him was, 'Where's the fun in your life? What do you do that you really enjoy?' He was stumped. He didn't like his job much – it just paid well. He loved his wife and daughters, but he hardly ever saw them and when he did he was so stressed he couldn't enjoy them. The therapist asked when he last felt truly happy and my client admitted it was at university when he used to write music. So the therapist asked, 'Why don't you do it now?' It was a simple enough question, but it floored my client. He had forgotten one of the simplest rules in life: do something you enjoy. It wasn't as simple as writing a few songs and having his depression cured, but over time, he felt his depression lift. With my help he started eating Clean & Lean. Because he was so stressed we reduced his exercise time (too much exercise – especially cardio – can actually raise stress levels and make anxiety worse). He's now much happier and loves spending time with his family. He still finds work stressful, but he can cope just fine.

EAT YOUR WAY TO BEING LESS STRESSED

Here's a list of foods that will help to reduce your stress levels.

1. KIWI FRUITS

Kiwi fruits give you a huge hit of vitamin C (as do oranges, kale, red, yellow and orange peppers, broccoli and strawberries) and can help reduce levels of stress hormones in the blood, according to a study from Indiana University East in America. Vitamins will provide more energy to help combat stress, while the folate can help to enhance your mood.

2. OMEGA-3 FATTY ACIDS

These are found in oily fish like salmon and fresh tuna. A study from Ohio State University in the US found that foods rich in omega-3s could help to decrease anxiety. This is because omega-3s reduce the level of cytokines, compounds whose production is increased with stress.

3. OATMEAL

Oatmeal and other complex carbohydrate-rich foods increase serotonin levels in the brain, according to another study from Indiana University East. Serotonin is a neurotransmitter that can help promote calmness.

4. SPINACH

This dark green vegetable is rich in vitamin C and contains high levels of magnesium. According to studies, low magnesium levels can cause headaches and fatigue, which can put extra stress on your body. Eating a diet rich in magnesium can help ward off stress and boost energy levels. Spinach is also a great source of iron which increases energy levels (which are often run down when we're stressed).

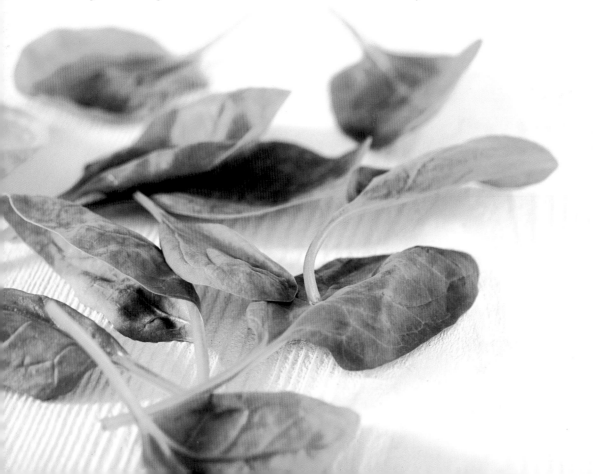

5. WALNUTS

These nuts are high in fibre, antioxidants and unsaturated fatty acids, all of which help to lower cholesterol and blood pressure during stressful situations. US researchers at Penn State University found a connection between walnut consumption and the increased ability of your body to handle stress.

6. PISTACHIO NUTS

According to a study conducted at Pennsylvania State University, eating pistachio nuts may reduce the body's response to life's everyday stresses. The nuts help lower blood pressure and heart rate in difficult situations.

7. TURKEY

Turkey is high in L-tryptophan – an amino acid that the body uses to release the feel-good hormone serotonin. A study from the University of Texas found that regularly eating turkey can help reduce stress levels.

8. SWEET POTATOES

These tasty potatoes can be stress-reducing because they satisfy the urge we get for carbohydrates and sweets when we feel stressed. Research at the University of Vienna says sweet potatoes also help to control blood sugar, therefore reducing stress levels. They contain more fibre and vitamins than regular white potatoes, too – and I actually prefer them.

*top tip

Try a yoga class this week and take three big, deep breaths now – you'll feel better, I promise.

FOODS THAT INCREASE STRESS

Just as the foods in the previous top ten – and many more Clean & Lean foods described in this book – can help your stress levels, there are others that can stress out your body and make you feel worse. Ironically, they tend to be the things you reach for when you feel burnt out, but it's really important you avoid these or cut back on them when you're wound up.

∗ **Caffeine** can stress out your system by constantly flooding your body with the fat-storing hormone cortisol, as I explained in Chapter 1, so just stick to one or two cups of coffee a day.

∗ **Alcohol** stimulates your poor, overworked adrenal glands even further. If you have a stressful life and you drink a lot, your adrenal glands will be exhausted and you'll eventually burn out. So please go easy on alcohol to give them a chance to recover. Alcohol is also full of sugar which makes you toxic and fat. People mistakenly think it will help them unwind after a hard day, but it has the opposite effect – it just stresses your whole system further. If you feel very stressed, avoid alcohol altogether until you feel better.

∗ **Sweets and sugary snacks** give you a quick burst of energy, but then they cause your blood-sugar levels to crash, leaving you feeling sluggish, stressed and with poor concentration. Don't make your system more stressed by jumping on the sugar rollercoaster.

∗ **Processed foods** are full of so much junk they deplete the levels of vitamins and minerals in your body that are vital for fighting stress. Keep yourself powered up and strong with Clean & Lean foods.

∗ **Junk food** that is high in bad fats (burgers, chips, kebabs, etc.) has been shown in several studies to lower concentration levels and increase stress.

∗ **Salty foods** increase your blood pressure which makes you more prone to stress. In particular, avoid processed meats like ham and bacon, crisps, salted nuts and processed foods which are stuffed with salt.

DON'T STRESS EAT

The way you eat is almost as important as what you eat. You can eat healthy food and exercise regularly, but if you feel constantly stressed, you'll never be truly Clean & Lean because stress itself is so toxic.

One of the best things you can do for your body – and I tell this to all my clients – is to learn how to chew properly. Chewing is the cornerstone of healthy eating. A salad becomes so much healthier when you chew it properly. Why? Because chewing food releases all the vitamins and minerals contained in the food. Chewing also produces saliva and breaks down food so your digestive system is ready for it. Well-digested food results in a flat stomach. Poorly digested food sits and ferments in your gut leaving you bloated, gassy and feeling sluggish and leading to long-term problems. Plus, your body won't get all the nutrients it needs to stay strong. So every time you eat, chew each mouthful of food ten, twenty, even thirty times. It will take a bit of getting used to, but you'll notice your stomach looks flatter and you'll feel better for it.

Also, don't shovel down food while you're watching TV or rushing to meet a deadline: firstly, you won't pay attention to what you're eating, so your brain won't register you're full (causing you to overeat); and secondly, you won't chew it properly (causing gas and bloating – see above). Instead, set aside ten minutes (at least) to sit down and focus on your food. Taste it, savour it, be grateful for it, chew it properly and your brain will register it more efficiently, so you'll stay fuller for longer and the meal will nourish you, making you stronger.

BREATHE BETTER

When we're stressed we take short, shallow breaths that make us even more stressed. When you feel yourself getting wound up, take a deep breath through your nose – the kind of breath that puffs up your chest because it's so full of air – and right down to your belly. Exhale through your mouth – enough to make your upper chest and shoulders sort of 'collapse' with relief. Do this three or four times and your stress levels will fall.

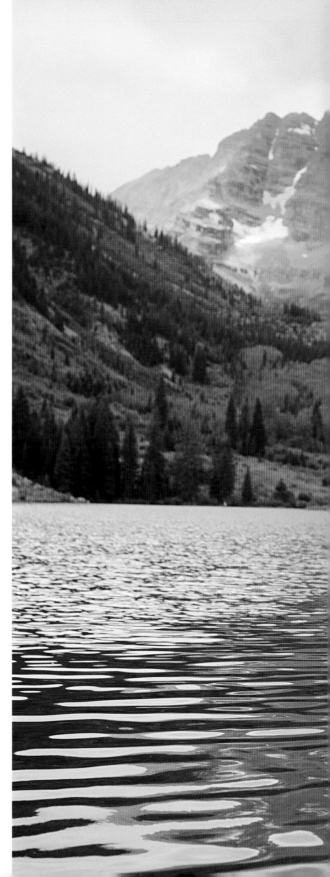

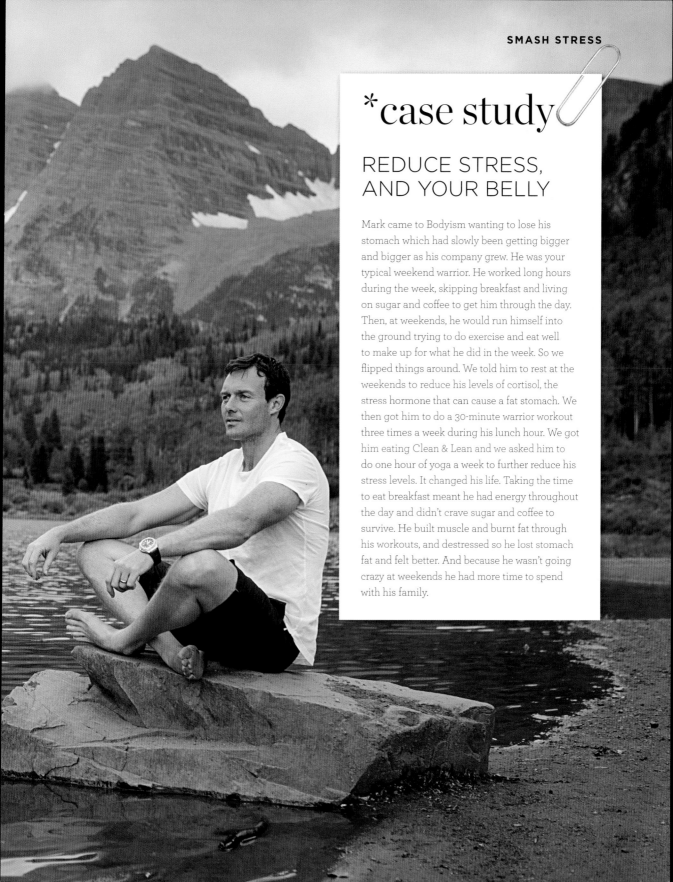

*case study

REDUCE STRESS, AND YOUR BELLY

Mark came to Bodyism wanting to lose his stomach which had slowly been getting bigger and bigger as his company grew. He was your typical weekend warrior. He worked long hours during the week, skipping breakfast and living on sugar and coffee to get him through the day. Then, at weekends, he would run himself into the ground trying to do exercise and eat well to make up for what he did in the week. So we flipped things around. We told him to rest at the weekends to reduce his levels of cortisol, the stress hormone that can cause a fat stomach. We then got him to do a 30-minute warrior workout three times a week during his lunch hour. We got him eating Clean & Lean and we asked him to do one hour of yoga a week to further reduce his stress levels. It changed his life. Taking the time to eat breakfast meant he had energy throughout the day and didn't crave sugar and coffee to survive. He built muscle and burnt fat through his workouts, and destressed so he lost stomach fat and felt better. And because he wasn't going crazy at weekends he had more time to spend with his family.

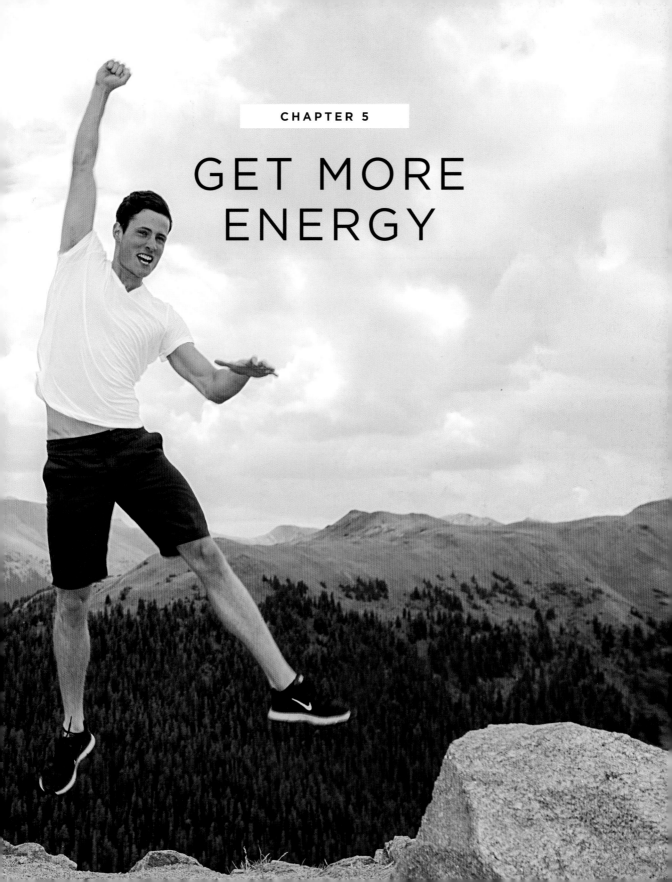

CHAPTER 5

GET MORE ENERGY

GET INSTANT ENERGY

Low energy levels often go hand in hand with being overweight, not getting enough sleep and feeling stressed all the time. If you're overweight and eating processed, nutritionally void food, your body isn't being nourished by the vitamins and minerals it needs to keep you energised. Eating nutrient-dense food will keep you fuller for longer and also help you eat less junk. As I explained in the previous chapter, if you're stressed, your adrenal glands will be overworked, which leads to tiredness. And stress and a bad diet can disrupt your sleep, which makes you even more tired. All these things feed off each other, keeping you stuck in a cycle of tiredness and often depression.

Some studies also suggest that low energy levels in men are linked to declining testosterone levels. As men age, their testosterone levels fall naturally which can make them prone to irritability (hence the grumpy old man stereotype) and tiredness. However, things like obesity, not enough good fat (see below) and too much alcohol can also lower testosterone levels in younger men, which, in turn, lowers their energy levels. Baldness and man boobs are often signs of low testosterone levels, too. Many things can increase testosterone levels, including exercise, reduced alcohol intake and a healthy diet. Plenty of good fat has been shown to boost testosterone levels, which is why I've included information about fat in this chapter.

MAYBE YOU NEED MORE GOOD FAT

Do you suffer from the following? If so, eat more fat!

* Inability to concentrate
* Sluggishness
* A mid-afternoon energy drop
* Difficulty waking up in the morning
* A feeling of lethargy and fatigue
* An over-reliance on coffee or sugary foods to perk you up throughout the day

DON'T BE AFRAID OF FAT

If you've tried dieting in the past, you may have cut out all types of fat, but here's why you shouldn't: good fat (by which I mean the type found in foods like nuts, seeds, oils, lean meat, fish, seafood and avocados, not the type found in oily pizzas or fatty meats) prevents you from overeating and tells your brain when to stop eating. This is why fat-phobic dieters are hungry all the time (and tired and miserable). There's something in good fat that switches on your brain's 'full' signals, and studies show that people who eat good fat every day are leaner than those who don't. It also helps you burn fat and means the body can function at its athletic best. Believe me guys, this is what you want. So have some good fat with every single meal and snack: if you have fruit, have a few almonds or walnuts at the same time; if you have a salad, add some avocado or olive oil. Fat slows the rate at which sugar hits your blood and this keeps your blood-sugar levels steady, which keeps you energised.

Good fat also burns fat around your waist and stomach and can give you a 6-pack. Essential fatty acids (essential because your body does not produce them) – found in oily fish like salmon, olive oil, nuts and so on – help shift fat out of the fat cells and into the bloodstream where it can be worked off by the body. Studies also show that these fatty acids help the body burn fat around your midriff. So choose butter over margarine (it's so full of flavour you'll only need a little bit) and olive oil over low-fat (i.e. high-sugar) salad dressings.

Fat also helps your body absorb vitamins and minerals better. Studies show that the vitamins in many vegetables are fat-soluble – meaning your body absorbs them more efficiently if they're eaten with fat. So always have a little olive oil, organic butter or goats' cheese with your vegetables. As I explained earlier – a body full of nutrients doesn't feel as tired, so remembering to add fat to your meals will really fire you up.

Good fat also helps cushion your joints from wear and tear, so if you exercise regularly, good fat will help prevent injuries. Finally, good fat keeps you alert and improves your concentration.

THE FACTS ABOUT CHOLESTEROL

There are two types of cholesterol – one good and one bad. LDL (Low Density Lipoprotein) is 'bad' cholesterol. It can build up in your arteries, which feed blood to your heart and brain. Over time it forms a hard plaque that narrows your arteries (known as atherosclerosis). If an artery becomes too narrow, a clot can form and a heart attack or stroke may follow. Eating foods high in saturated fat can raise bad cholesterol levels, and these include fatty cuts of meat like sausage pies, cakes and biscuits. Fibre helps sweep bad cholesterol out of your system, and these include fruits, vegetables, lentils, chickpeas and beans. Exercise also helps lower bad cholesterol.

HDL (High Density Lipoprotein) is 'good' cholesterol. HDL carry bad cholesterol away from the arteries to the liver, where it's processed from the body. HDL also removes plaque from bad cholesterol from the arteries, which reduces harmful build ups. Foods high in unsaturated fat can help lower bad cholesterol levels, like oily fish, nuts and seeds.

FATS TO AVOID

Here's my guide to the fats you should be avoiding:

✳ Anything with a crust (pies, quiches, etc.)
✳ Pizza – cheap frozen ones with processed ham and cheese toppings are the worst; if you love pizza, make one yourself using lots of lovely fresh tomato sauce, fresh basil and plenty of good-quality, unprocessed protein like chicken or prawns (or order one from a good restaurant and ask for extra protein)
✳ Ready meals – they nearly all contain too much saturated fat
✳ Shop-bought cakes, biscuits and muffins – they're full of toxic, cheap fat; if you love this kind of thing, make it yourself at home or buy it fresh from a local baker or farmer's market
✳ Anything described as deep-fried, sautéed or breaded
✳ Any obvious fat on an animal product, such as the white rind on a slice of bacon
✳ Salad dressings – they're usually high in trans fats. Add olive oil to your salad instead

WHY YOU SHOULD TAKE FAT SUPPLEMENTS

I tell all my clients to take a fish oil (omega 3) supplement because they top up levels of essential fatty acids and encourage your body to burn fat (around your stomach and waist in particular), as well as boosting energy levels.

But how do you know the difference between a good and bad supplement? A good-quality one will dissolve thoroughly if you leave it in a glass of room-temperature water overnight, whereas a cheap, poor-quality one won't. And you should also store your fish oils in the fridge to keep them good.

THE MANY FACES OF FAT

Good fat is monounsaturated fat and, as I've said, it's found mainly in nuts, avocados and olive oil. It helps lower bad cholesterol and reduces overall body fat by increasing your metabolism. Polyunsaturated fat – found mainly in fish and seafood – also lowers bad cholesterol levels.

Saturated fat should only be enjoyed occasionally, although it's not as bad as trans fats (see p. 21) which should be cut out of your diet entirely. Saturated fat raises bad cholesterol levels and is found mainly in non-organic animal products like meat and full-fat dairy. I love red meat which contains saturated fat and, as I've said, you can enjoy it occasionally, but don't overdo it. The same also goes for dairy. Enjoy it by all means but, when you do, make sure it is organic and full-fat and rotate it with dairy alternatives, like almond milk.

FAT-BURNING NUTS AND SEEDS

A handful of any of the below make a great quick snack

* Almonds
* Pecans
* Walnuts
* Brazil nuts
* Pistachios
* Macadamias
* Cashews
* Chestnuts
* Sesame seeds
* Peanuts
* Sunflower seeds
* Pumpkin seeds
* Linseed (ground only)

FAT-BURNING FISH

Try to eat at least three portions a week (see fromfishtofork.com for sustainable sources)

* Salmon
* Trout
* Pilchards
* Mackerel
* Anchovies
* Herrings
* Sardines
* Kippers
* Whitebait
* Tuna (go for fresh steaks or the kind you can buy in glass jars – mainly available in health-food shops or independent delis)
* Swordfish

FAT-BLITZING OILS

When cooking on a medium heat

* Extra-virgin olive oil
* Macadamia nut oil
* Avocado oil

When cooking on a high heat

* Ghee oil
* Coconut oil

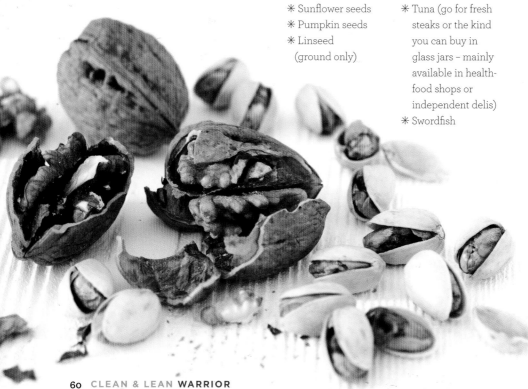

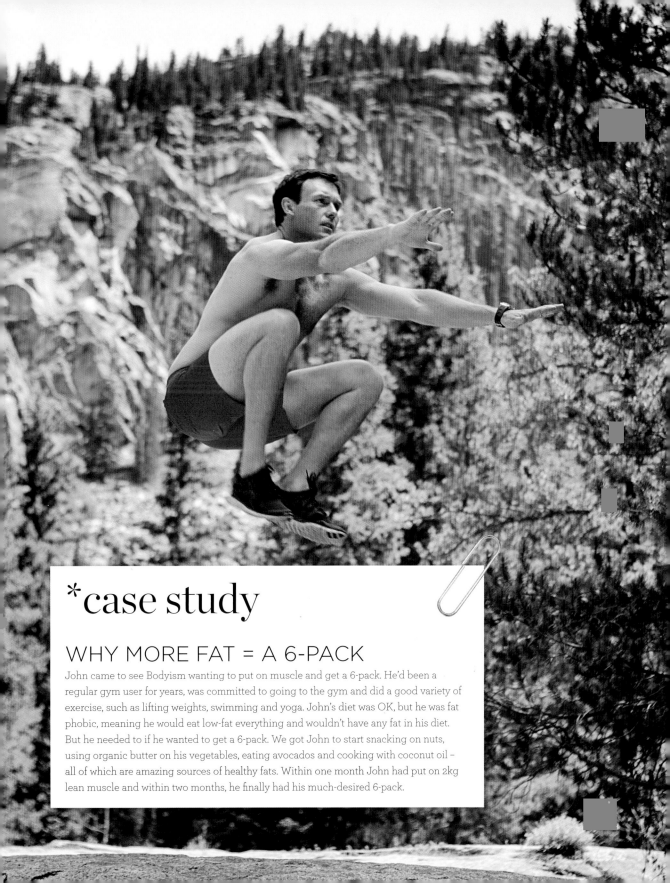

*case study

WHY MORE FAT = A 6-PACK

John came to see Bodyism wanting to put on muscle and get a 6-pack. He'd been a regular gym user for years, was committed to going to the gym and did a good variety of exercise, such as lifting weights, swimming and yoga. John's diet was OK, but he was fat phobic, meaning he would eat low-fat everything and wouldn't have any fat in his diet. But he needed to if he wanted to get a 6-pack. We got John to start snacking on nuts, using organic butter on his vegetables, eating avocados and cooking with coconut oil – all of which are amazing sources of healthy fats. Within one month John had put on 2kg lean muscle and within two months, he finally had his much-desired 6-pack.

BAD, BETTER AND BEST GUIDE TO

BAD	BETTER	BEST
Vegetable oil	Rapeseed oil	Organic extra-virgin coconut oil (this isn't broken down under high heat)
Shop-bought salad dressing	Extra-virgin olive oil	Organic cold-pressed extra-virgin olive oil
Margarine	Regular butter	Unsalted raw butter
Regular cow's butter	Organic cow's butter	Organic goat's butter
Doughnuts – packed with fat, sugar and additives	Muffin from a health-food store – it may contain some fibre and fruit (and satisfy your sweet craving), but it's still full of fat and sugar	Fruit and nuts – the perfect mix of fat and good sugar to satisfy your sweet craving and help fill you up
Croissant – soaked in bad, cheap fats (one that's freshly made from a bakery is better than a shop-bought one because at least it will contain fewer additives and preservatives)	Muffin from health-food store – see above	Raw vegetables with just a little organic hummus – loads of fibre, vitamins and minerals
Bacon – full of nitrates which drag nutrients from your body, including essential vitamins A, C and E	Pre-sliced gammon/ham – salty and contains additives	Organic ham off the bone. Good, clean protein
Chips or crisps – the thinner they are, the fewer nutrients and more bad fats they contain	Salted unroasted nuts – a much better alternative for satisfying hunger	Raw organic unsalted nuts – good, clean protein
Fried chicken from a high-street restaurant – poor-quality meat wrapped in a layer of lard	Barbecue chicken with salad – better-quality protein and a lot less fat. Just take off the skin to reduce fat further	Turkey breast and super greens – a very lean meat that helps you sleep and improves energy levels the next day
Burger and fries – high-street burger buns are so full of sugar they should be called cakes. And the beef is poor quality	Burger and salad – breadless means less sugar and more room for the energy-boosting nutrients from the salad	Lean beef stir-fry with loads of vegetables – quick and delicious. Feeds your muscles and burns fat
Frozen pizza	Pizza from a good Italian restaurant	Homemade pizza

EATING THE RIGHT FAT

BAD	BETTER	BEST
Deep-fried fish – clogs up your heart, makes you tired and gives you a fat belly	Pan-fried fish and salad – if you're in a restaurant, always ask for your fish to be pan-fried or grilled	Grilled fish and a green salad. If you add olive oil to the salad, this is the perfect meal – best there is
Sausage rolls – poor-quality meat wrapped in buttered pastry	Lamb or chicken kebab with salad	Lamb or chicken with salad
Sausage	Organic sausage	Organic steak
Scrambled or fried eggs	Poached or boiled eggs	Organic or free-range poached or boiled eggs
Tinned meat	Fresh meat	Fresh organic meat
Battered or crumbed fish	Fresh farmed fish	Wild/organic fish
Packaged sliced ham	Ham off the bone	Organic ham off the bone
Malibu and cola – sugar with more sugar, plus caffeine and alcohol	Malibu and pineapple juice – some natural sugars, but still a fat bomb	Vodka with a fruit smoothie – clean spirit with plenty of nutrients and a little bit of fibre. Sip it slowly and enjoy the taste
Processed cheese slices	Block of supermarket cheese	Organic goat's cheese – the least processed of all cheeses
Tinned tuna	Tinned mackerel	Line-caught tinned sardines
Tinned salmon	Farmed smoked salmon	Organic smoked salmon

ENERGY BOOSTERS

It's pretty easy to improve your energy levels by eating Clean & Lean and regularly following the exercises in Chapter 8. There are also certain foods that boost flagging energy levels. So if you always feel weary and struggle to get out of bed in the mornings, try including the following in your diet:

Nuts

According to a recent US study, almonds, cashews and hazelnuts in particular can boost your energy levels thanks to their magnesium.

Lentils

As well as clearing out your digestive system (a healthy digestion boosts your energy levels, which is why constipation leaves you feeling so tired), lentils are a good source of the mineral molybdenum, which can keep your energy levels high.

Spinach

Thanks to the fact it's full of potassium, iron and magnesium it helps to boost energy. Eat it as raw as possible to retain all the goodness. If you want to cook it, lightly steam it rather than boiling it.

Green tea

This is a great source of caffeine, so it's a good early-morning pick-me-up. Studies show it also speeds up your metabolism. Have several cups a day in the place of coffee, but never have it after lunch – the caffeine will make it hard to fall asleep.

Eggs

One of my favourite foods, these are full of an energy-improving mix of selenium, amino acids and vitamins. Have them for breakfast to fire you up. They're also good for creating lean muscle mass and they keep you full for hours.

SLEEP YOURSELF STRONGER

Sleep is a vital part of the Clean & Lean regime. A decent amount of sleep leaves you stronger, leaner and more energised. A lack of sleep lowers your immunity, makes you crave fatty and sugary foods and it ages your body. In terms of how many hours you need, aim for seven or eight, although generally I tell clients to stick to an amount of time that suits them. Some of us can get by on five or six hours a night while others need eight or nine. Here's how to improve your sleep:

1 SET THE SCENE
One of the biggest reasons for a bad night's sleep is your pre-bed routine. Your mind and body need to wind down if you want to get into a proper sleep, which means no TV, no iPad, no mobile or laptop and no arguing with your partner before bed. If you're worried about something, write it down and promise yourself you'll deal with it tomorrow.

An hour before you plan to go to bed, turn off all your electronic equipment and read a good book, have sex (a fantastic stress-buster that also improves the quality of your sleep) or do some stretching (you'll find some stress-busting stretches in Chapter 7). Install blackout blinds in your bedroom because even a tiny bit of light in your bedroom can stop your melatonin levels from rising, which you need to induce sleep in the first place and to reach the deep, restorative sleep your body requires.

2 GO EASY ON EXERCISE IN THE EVENING
Studies show that too much vigorous exercise too late in the evening can keep you awake because it floods your body with hormones that keep you alert. However, gentle, mind-calming exercises such as Pilates or yoga have the opposite effect.

3 AVOID SLEEP-STEALING FOODS
What you eat and drink in the evening has a huge impact on how well you sleep. A heavy meal too close to bed will sit in your stomach overnight which may affect sleep. You should also avoid food or drink containing

caffeine at least eight hours before bed – that means the obvious ones like coffee, cola and tea, but also less obvious ones such as chocolate which can be full of caffeine. Alcohol also disrupts sleep. You may think you sleep well after a few beers, but you won't enter the proper deep stage of sleep that your body needs to stay strong and healthy. Nicotine found in cigarettes can keep you awake too, so if you're a smoker, try to have your last one well before bed or, better still, quit.

4 EAT SLEEP-INDUCING FOODS

Studies show that if you eat foods rich in tryptophan during the day, you'll sleep better that night. Tryptophan-rich foods include nuts, beans, fish, cheese and eggs, so try to eat at least one of them every day. For your evening meal eat foods that release serotonin (the feel-good hormone), such as sweet potatoes, bananas and turkey.

5 SUPPLEMENTS

Herbs such as valerian and camomile and vitamins including magnesium and B6 are natural sedatives. Valerian has been used for centuries to improve sleep, and reduce stress and anxiety (it's thought to have a gentle tranquilising effect on the central nervous system). I also invented Body Serenity, which is the best thing in the world for sleep. Go to bodyism.com.

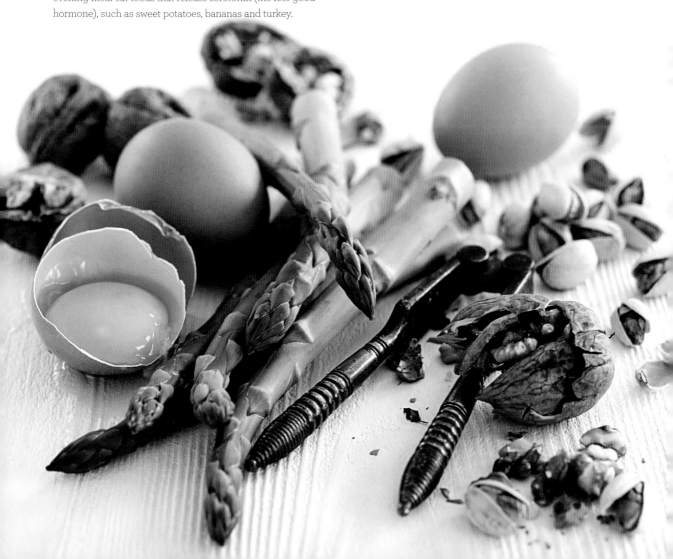

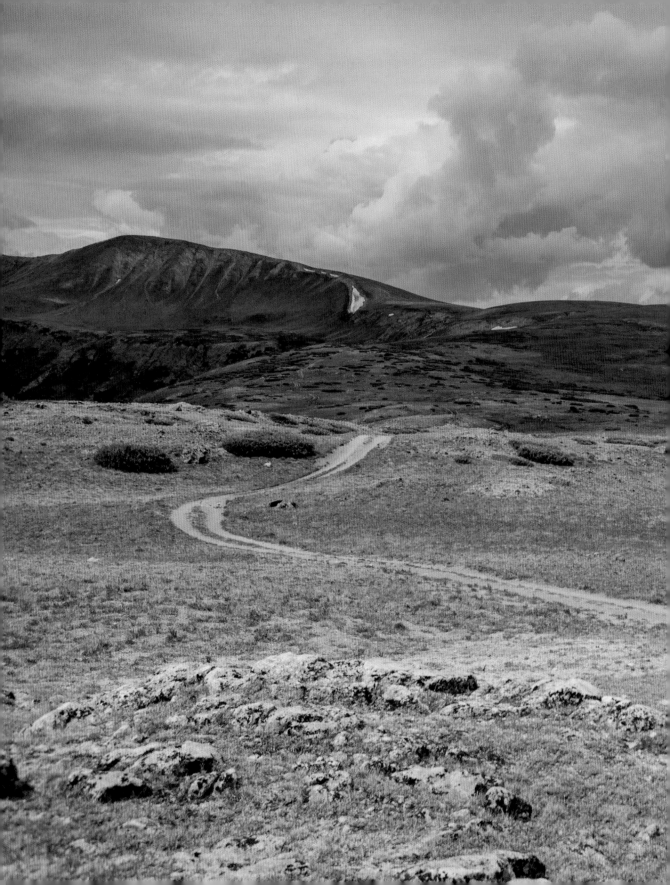

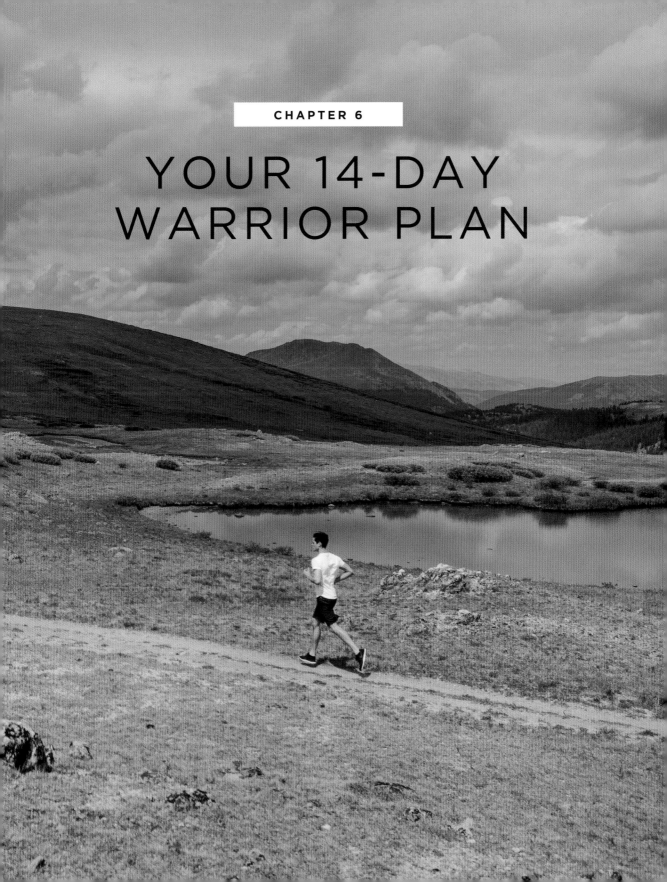

CHAPTER 6

YOUR 14-DAY WARRIOR PLAN

YOUR 14-DAY WARRIOR BLUEPRINT

When you feel ready, start this 14-day programme. It's often good to begin on a weekend as then you have more time and, by Monday, you're already into your routine.

You can swap meals around (have Day 1 breakfast on Day 2, for example), but try to stick to the plan as much as possible. You shouldn't feel hungry but, if you do, just increase your green vegetable and protein portions and make sure you're drinking enough water (at least 2–3 litres of still, filtered water a day). Where possible, go for organic ingredients but, if that's tricky, don't worry – just do the best you can and don't let anything get in your way. When you have followed this 14-day plan and repeated it a few times, go to our website (cleanandlean.com) for new programmes to add variety. However, for now, this is an excellent place to start. Be a man – get it done no matter what!

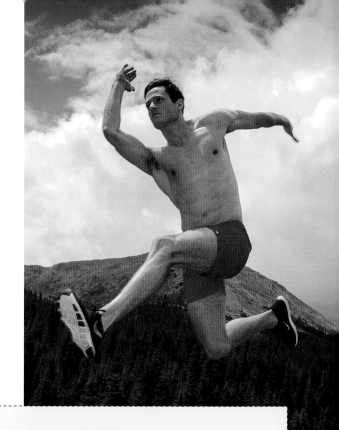

MEN'S 14-DAY WARRIOR BLUEPRINT

Day 1
A.M. Upper Body Workout (pp. 85–88)
P.M. 20 min Blast with Cardio (pp. 98–103)

Day 2
Lower Body Workout (pp. 89–93)

Day 3
A.M. Ab Workout (pp. 94–97)
P.M. 20 min Blast with Cardio (pp. 98–103)

Day 4
Rest Day

Day 5
A.M. Upper Body Workout (pp. 85–88)
P.M. 20 min Blast with Cardio (pp. 98–103)

Day 6
Lower Body Workout (pp. 89–93)

Day 7
A.M. Ab Workout (pp. 94–97)
P.M. 20 min Blast with Cardio (pp. 98–103)

Day 8
Rest Day

Day 9
A.M. Upper Body Workout (pp. 85–88)
P.M. 20 min Blast with Cardio (pp. 98–103)

Day 10
Lower Body Workout (pp. 89–93)

Day 11
A.M. Ab Workout (pp. 94–97)
P.M. 20 min Blast with Cardio (pp. 98–103)

Day 12
Rest Day

Day 13
A.M. Upper Body Workout (pp. 85–88)
P.M. 20 min Blast with Cardio (pp. 98–103)

Day 14
A.M. Lower Body Workout (pp. 89–93)
P.M. 20 min Blast with Cardio (pp. 98–103)

THE PROGRAMMES

PROGRAMME 1

UPPER BODY WORKOUT

Perform each exercise one after the other with a 30-second rest between each exercise. Perform each circuit 4 times and rest for 90 seconds between circuits.

✳ Reverse Grip Bicep Curl to Shoulder Press (p. 85)
4 x 15 reps/ 30-second rest

✳ Bent Over Row Reverse Grip (p. 86)
4 x 15 reps/ 30-second rest

✳ Single Arm Shoulder Press (p. 87)
4 x 10 each side/ 30-second rest

✳ Bent Over Row Underhand Grip (p. 88)
4 x 15 reps/ 90-second rest

PROGRAMME 2

LOWER BODY WORKOUT

Perform each exercise one after the other with a 30-second rest between each exercise. Perform each circuit 4 times and rest for 90 seconds between circuits.

✳ Squat Press (p. 89)
4 x 15 reps/ 30-second rest

✳ Ab Lunge with Twist (p. 90)
4 x 10 each side/ 30-second rest

✳ Overhead Lunge (p. 91)
4 x 10 each leg/ 30-second rest

✳ Lunge get up with Log (pp. 92–93)
4 x 10 each leg/ 90-second rest

PROGRAMME 3

AB WORKOUT

Perform each exercise one after the other with a 30-second rest between each exercise. Perform each circuit 5 times and rest for 90 seconds between circuits.

✳ Wood chop (p. 94)
5 x 10 each side/ 30-second rest

✳ Ab Lunge with Twist (p. 95)
5 x 10 each leg/ 30-second rest

✳ Kayak Sit up (pp. 96–97)
5 x 40 twists (20 each side)/ 90-second rest

PROGRAMME 4

20-MIN BLAST WITH CARDIO

Perform each exercise one after the other with a 15-second rest between each exercise. Perform each circuit 5 times and rest for 60 seconds between circuits.

✳ Burpee (pp. 98–99)
5 x 30 seconds / 15-second rest

✳ Disco Lunge (p. 100)
5 x 30 seconds / 15-second rest

✳ Spiderman Push Up (p. 101)
5 x 30 seconds / 15-second rest

✳ Mountain Climbers (pp. 102–103)
5 x 30 seconds / 60-second rest

*top tip

For more programmes, please go online to cleanandlean.com or bodyism.com.

	DAY 1	DAY 2	DAY 3
WAKING UP	1 glass of filtered water with a fresh squeeze of lemon or lime and a pinch of Himalayan salt	1 glass of filtered water with a fresh squeeze of lemon or lime and a pinch of Himalayan salt	1 glass of filtered water with a fresh squeeze of lemon or lime and a pinch of Himalayan salt
BREAKFAST	200–300g white fish or beef with 1 whole avocado and 8–10 grilled asparagus spears with scrambled eggs	2 grilled mackerel fillets or 2 grilled chicken breasts with 100g cooked spinach and 1 tablespoon hummus (p. 132)	2–3 poached eggs with 200g smoked salmon or 2 grilled turkey breasts with 200g cooked kale
SNACK	6–8 raw carrot sticks with 2 teaspoons Brazil Nut Butter	1–2 Grilled Turkey and Vegetable Skewers	110g Bodyism Guacamole (p. 132) with 6–8 red pepper wedges
LUNCH	Clean & Lean Turkey Lettuce Wraps (p. 128)	grilled prawns over a mixed green salad with avocado and pumpkin seeds	Clean & Lean Superfood Chicken Salad (p. 131)
SNACK	1–2 Grilled Chicken and Mushroom Skewers	6–8 cucumber sticks with 2 teaspoons Hazelnut Butter	Clean & Lean Prawn Lettuce Wraps (p. 128)
DINNER	2 grilled turkey breasts with 225–450g cooked broccoli	1 fillet grilled white fish with 10 grilled asparagus spears and a handful of shaved almonds	Chicken Stir Fry with Coconut Oil and Mixed Vegetables

HOW MUCH IS 100G?

If you don't have scales to weigh your portions, here's a rough guide to the measurements given in the 14-day plan above:

100g chicken = two thirds the size of a regular breast or the palm of your hand (minus fingers)

100g smoked salmon = the size of your outstretched hand (including fingers)

100g beef fillet = the size of a tennis ball

*top tip

Many of the dishes here are included in the recipe chapter (pp. 116–153). Find others on our website, cleanandlean.com.

DAY 4	DAY 5	DAY 6	DAY 7
1 glass of filtered water with a fresh squeeze of lemon or lime and a pinch of Himalayan salt	1 glass of filtered water with a fresh squeeze of lemon or lime and a pinch of Himalayan salt	1 glass of filtered water with a fresh squeeze of lemon or lime and a pinch of Himalayan salt	1 glass of filtered water with a fresh squeeze of lemon or lime and a pinch of Himalayan salt
Super Clean & Lean Breakfast (p. 123)	3-egg omelette with 2 grilled mackerel fillets or 2 grilled chicken breasts, 200g cooked spinach and chopped tomatoes	200g smoked salmon or 2 grilled turkey breasts with 200g cooked kale, 1 whole avocado and tomato salsa	2-3 poached eggs with 2 grilled mackerel fillets or 2 grilled chicken breasts and 200g cooked spinach
1-2 Grilled Lamb and Pepper Skewers	6-8 cucumber sticks with 2 teaspoons Hazelnut Butter	1 - 2 Grilled Chicken and Mushroom Skewers	110g Bodyism Guacamole (p. 132) with 6-8 red pepper wedges
Greek Salad (p. 136) with 1-2 grilled chicken breasts (leave out the feta cheese)	Clean & Lean Chicken Lettuce Wraps (p. 128)	1-2 beef patties over a spinach salad with grilled tomatoes and chopped onions	Clean & Lean Superfood Chicken Salad (p. 131)
110g Bodyism Guacamole (p. 132) with 6-8 red bell pepper wedges	1-2 Grilled Lamb and Pepper Skewers	6-8 raw carrot sticks with 2 teaspoons Brazil Nut Butter	Clean & Lean Beef Lettuce Wraps (p. 128)
Bodyism Super Mince	1 fillet grilled white fish with 10 grilled asparagus spears and a handful of shaved almonds	Chicken Stir Fry with Coconut Oil and Mixed Vegetables	2 roasted turkey breasts with mixed green vegetables

*top tip

Stick this plan on your fridge as a constant reminder, then you won't be tempted to stray.

	DAY 8	DAY 9	DAY 10
WAKING UP	1 glass of filtered water with a fresh squeeze of lemon or lime and a pinch of Himalayan salt	1 glass of filtered water with a fresh squeeze of lemon or lime and a pinch of Himalayan salt	1 glass of filtered water with a fresh squeeze of lemon or lime and a pinch of Himalayan salt
BREAKFAST	2 grilled mackerel fillets or 2 grilled chicken breasts with 100g cooked spinach and 1 tablespoon hummus (p. 132)	spinach and tomato omelette with 1 whole sliced avocado	Super Clean & Lean Breakfast (p. 123)
SNACK	6–8 raw carrot sticks with 2 teaspoons Brazil Nut Butter	1–2 Grilled Turkey and Vegetable Skewers	110g Bodyism Guacamole (p. 132) with 6–8 red pepper wedges
LUNCH	Greek Salad (p. 136) with 1–2 grilled chicken breasts (leave out the feta cheese)	Clean & Lean Turkey Lettuce Wraps (p. 128)	Chicken Stir Fry with Coconut Oil and Mixed Vegetables
SNACK	1–2 Grilled Chicken & Mushroom Skewers	6–8 cucumber sticks with 2 teaspoons Hazelnut Butter	Clean & Lean Beef Lettuce Wraps (p. 128)
DINNER	1 fillet grilled white fish with 8–10 grilled asparagus spears and a handful of shaved almonds	Bodyism Super Mince	2 baked wild salmon fillets with 8–10 grilled asparagus spears and 200g cooked spinach

COOKING METHODS

You can choose your own cooking methods, but remember that you'll see quicker results if you steam or bake the vegetables and grill or bake the meat or fish. With vegetables, the less time you spend cooking them, the more nutrients will remain. Overcooked vegetables don't contain as many nutrients as lightly steamed ones.

STEAM/BLANCH/ GRILL

Steaming: One of the healthiest ways to cook as it retains nearly all the nutrients found in food and doesn't add any fat.

Blanching: This method keeps vegetables crisp and tender.

Grilling: This is a great way to cook meat and fish as the fat drips away, plus it tastes delicious.

DAY 11	DAY 12	DAY 13	DAY 14
1 glass of filtered water with a fresh squeeze of lemon or lime and a pinch of Himalayan salt	1 glass of filtered water with a fresh squeeze of lemon or lime and a pinch of Himalayan salt	1 glass of filtered water with a fresh squeeze of lemon or lime and a pinch of Himalayan salt	1 glass of filtered water with a fresh squeeze of lemon or lime and a pinch of Himalayan salt
2–3 poached eggs with 200g smoked salmon or 2 grilled turkey breasts with 200g cooked kale	2 grilled mackerel fillets or 2 grilled chicken breasts with 200g cooked spinach and 1 tablespoon hummus (p. 132)	200–300g white fish or beef with 1 whole avocado and 8–10 grilled asparagus spears with 110g Guacamole (p. 132)	200g smoked salmon or 2 grilled turkey breasts with 200g cooked kale, 1 whole avocado and tomato salsa
1–2 Grilled Lamb and Pepper Skewers	6–8 cucumber sticks with 2 teaspoons Hazelnut Butter	1 – 2 Grilled Chicken & Mushroom Skewers	6–8 raw carrot sticks with 2 teaspoons Brazil Nut Butter
1–2 beef patties over a spinach salad with grilled tomatoes and chopped onions	Clean & Lean Prawn Lettuce Wraps (p. 128)	grilled turkey pattie with a spinach salad, drizzled in extra-virgin olive oil	grilled prawns over a mixed green salad with avocado and pumpkin seeds
110g Bodyism Guacamole (p. 132) with 6–8 red pepper wedges	1–2 Grilled Turkey and Vegetable Skewers	6–8 carrot sticks with 2 teaspoons Brazil Nut Butter	Clean & Lean Beef Lettuce Wraps (p. 128)
Lemon-Roasted Chicken (p. 139) with 225–450g cooked broccoli	2–3 Grilled Lamb Chops with a Pecan and Kale Salad	Clean & Lean Beef Superfood Salad	2 caribbean chicken breasts with grilled broccoli and asparagus

*top tip

Save time and don't cook vegetables – you won't lose nutrients that way!

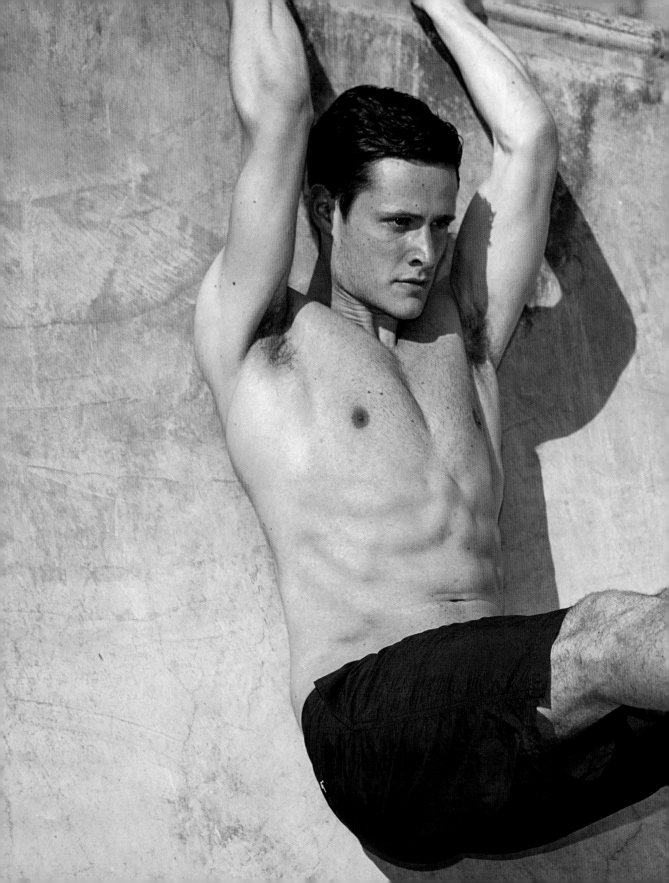

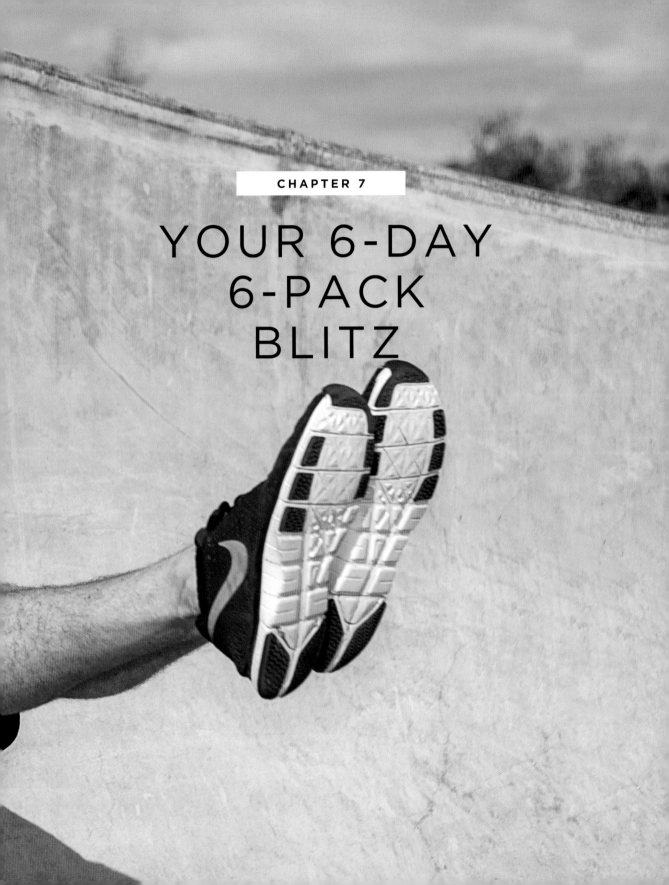

CHAPTER 7

YOUR 6-DAY 6-PACK BLITZ

YOUR 6-DAY
6-PACK BLITZ

OK, this is hardcore but I love it. I designed this with Lee Mullins, one of the best trainers in the world. He also happens to be one of my best friends. Listen to what we say here and I'm pretty sure you will see and feel a difference in your body. There are two exercise sessions each day as well as an eating programme for you to follow. If there are certain things you don't like then just substitute them for something else on the plan. If you don't want to stink the office out with fish, then swap the fish lunch for a Clean & Lean wrap or whatever you feel like at the time. OK, good luck and enjoy!

RULES OF THE
6-DAY 6-PACK
BLITZ

✳ Limit your salt intake – it holds on to water, which causes tummy bloating.

✳ No spicy herbs – chilli inflames the gut wall and makes it stick out.

✳ Water only – unlike the 14-day plan where you can have coffee every day, here you can't. The only caffeine you can have is in green tea, which is so full of antioxidants it helps reduce stress on the body (remember: stress = a fat stomach).

✳ Limit your fat intake, and I recommend taking a Clean & Lean fish oil capsule at each meal.

✳ All food has to be steamed, baked or grilled. Boring, but brilliantly effective in six days.

✳ You need to drink at least 2–3 litres of still filtered water a day. Along with all the fibre you're having, this will sweep through your system, cleaning out your bowels and giving a flatter, leaner stomach.

✳ Talking of fibre, you'll need lots of it – it rids the body of toxins and foreign oestrogen (from medication, the environment, etc., leading to moobs, those 'man boobs' again!).

The green vegetables in this 6-day 6-pack blitz have been specifically chosen to help your body become less acidic (remember, less acid = a flatter stomach). This helps your body burn fat faster (especially around the middle). Plus it means fewer toxins in your system, which benefits your waist, stomach, overall health and overall appearance (better skin, hair, etc.). As you won't be eating any complex carbs (such as bread, pasta, rice) your body will constantly be burning fat.

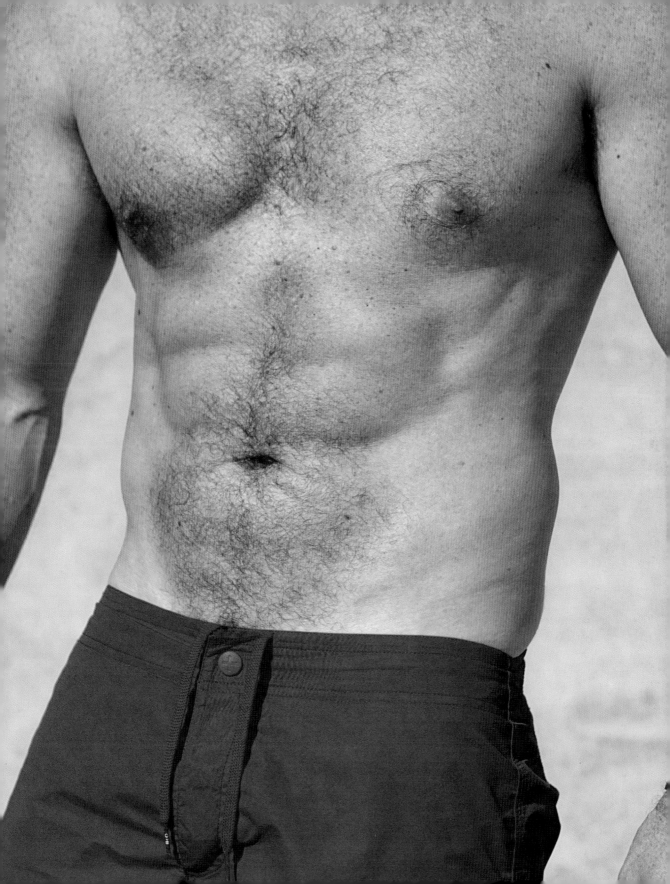

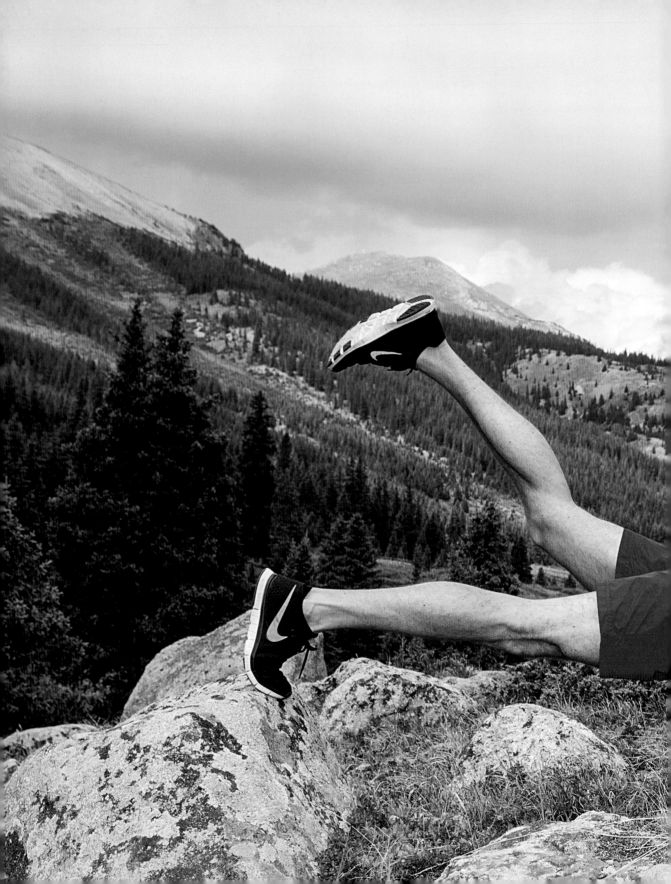

MEN'S 6-DAY 6-PACK WARRIOR WORKOUT

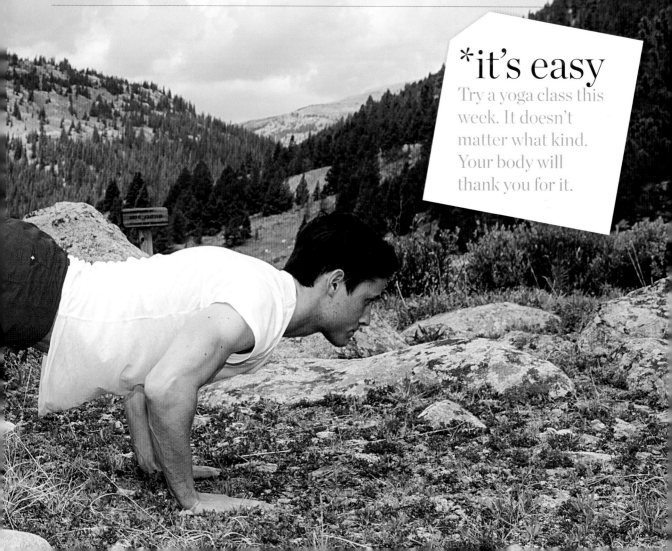

DAY 1	DAY 2	DAY 3	DAY 4	DAY 5	DAY 6
Morning Upper Body Workout (pp. 85–88)	**Morning** Lower Body Workout (pp. 89–93)	**Morning** Upper Body Workout (pp. 85–88)	**Morning** Lower Body Workout (pp. 89–93)	**Morning** Upper Body Workout (pp. 85–88)	**Morning** Lower Body Workout (pp. 89–93)
Evening Ab Workout (pp. 94–97)	**Evening** 20 min Blast with Cardio (pp. 98–103)	**Evening** Ab Workout (pp. 94–97)	**Evening** 20 min Blast with Cardio (pp. 98–103)	**Evening** Ab Workout (pp. 94–97)	**Evening** 20 min Blast with Cardio (pp. 98–103)

*it's easy
Try a yoga class this week. It doesn't matter what kind. Your body will thank you for it.

	DAY 1	DAY 2	DAY 3
WAKING UP	1 glass of filtered water with a fresh squeeze of lemon or lime and a pinch of Himalayan salt	1 glass of filtered water with a fresh squeeze of lemon or lime and a pinch of Himalayan salt	1 glass of filtered water with a fresh squeeze of lemon or lime and a pinch of Himalayan salt
BREAKFAST	200–300g grilled white fish or beef with 1 whole avocado and 8–10 grilled asparagus spears	2 grilled mackerel fillets or grilled chicken breasts with 200g cooked spinach and a handful of mixed nuts	2–3 poached eggs with 200g smoked salmon or 2 grilled turkey breasts with 200g cooked kale and 1 whole avocado
SNACK	1–2 Grilled Lamb and Pepper Skewers	1–2 Grilled Turkey and Vegetable Skewers	1–2 Grilled Chicken and Mushroom Skewers
LUNCH	Greek Salad with 1–2 Grilled Chicken Breasts (leave out the feta cheese)	grilled prawns over a mixed green salad with avocado and pumpkin seeds	1–2 beef patties over a spinach salad with grilled tomatoes and chopped onions
SNACK	110g Bodyism Guacamole (p. 132) with 6–8 red pepper wedges	6–8 cucumber sticks with 2 teaspoons Hazelnut Butter	110g Bodyism Guacamole (p. 132) with 6–8 red pepper wedges
DINNER	2 grilled turkey breasts with 225–450g cooked broccoli	1 fillet grilled white fish with 8–10 grilled asparagus spears and a handful of shaved almonds	Chicken Stir Fry with Coconut Oil and Mixed Vegetables

*it's easy
The more nutrients your body consumes, the less hungry you'll feel.

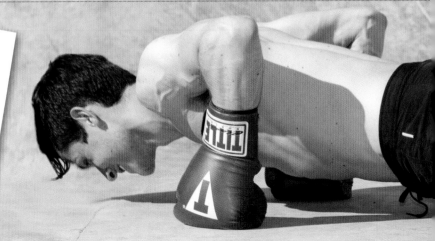

DAY 4

1 glass of filtered water with a fresh squeeze of lemon or lime and a pinch of Himalayan salt

200–300g grilled white fish or beef with 1 whole avocado and 8-10 grilled asparagus spears

1-2 Grilled Lamb and Pepper Skewers

Greek Salad with 1–2 Grilled Chicken Breasts (leave out the feta cheese)

6-8 cucumber sticks with 2 teaspoons Hazelnut Butter

grilled turkey pattie with a spinach salad, drizzled in extra-virgin olive oil

DAY 5

1 glass of filtered water with a fresh squeeze of lemon or lime and a pinch of Himalayan salt

2 grilled mackerel fillets or grilled chicken breasts with 200g cooked spinach and a handful of mixed nuts

1-2 Grilled Turkey and Vegetable Skewers

grilled prawns over a mixed green salad with avocado and pumpkin seeds

6-8 cucumber sticks with 2 teaspoons Hazelnut Butter

1 fillet grilled white fish with 8-10 grilled asparagus spears and a handful of shaved almonds

DAY 6

1 glass of filtered water with a fresh squeeze of lemon or lime and a pinch of Himalayan salt

2-3 poached eggs with 200g smoked salmon or 2 grilled turkey breasts with 200g cooked kale and 1 whole avocado

1-2 Grilled Chicken and Mushroom Skewers

1-2 beef patties over a spinach salad with grilled tomatoes and chopped onions

6-8 raw carrot sticks with 2 teaspoons Brazil Nut Butter

Lemon-Roasted Chicken (p. 139) with 225–450g cooked broccoli

PROTEIN SWAP

These menu plans are not intended to limit you in any way. Food is one of our main life sources and should be enjoyed, so feel free to swap any of the proteins if there is something else you prefer. If you don't like lamb, have beef instead. If you're vegetarian, opt for a non-meat source like eggs, beans, lentils etc. As for cheese, go for white cheese such as feta and goat's cheese. Avoid heavily processed cheeses that are bright yellow in colour or come in slices and go for the best quality organic cheese you can afford.

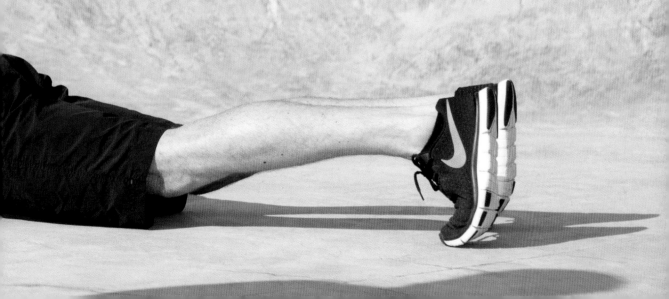

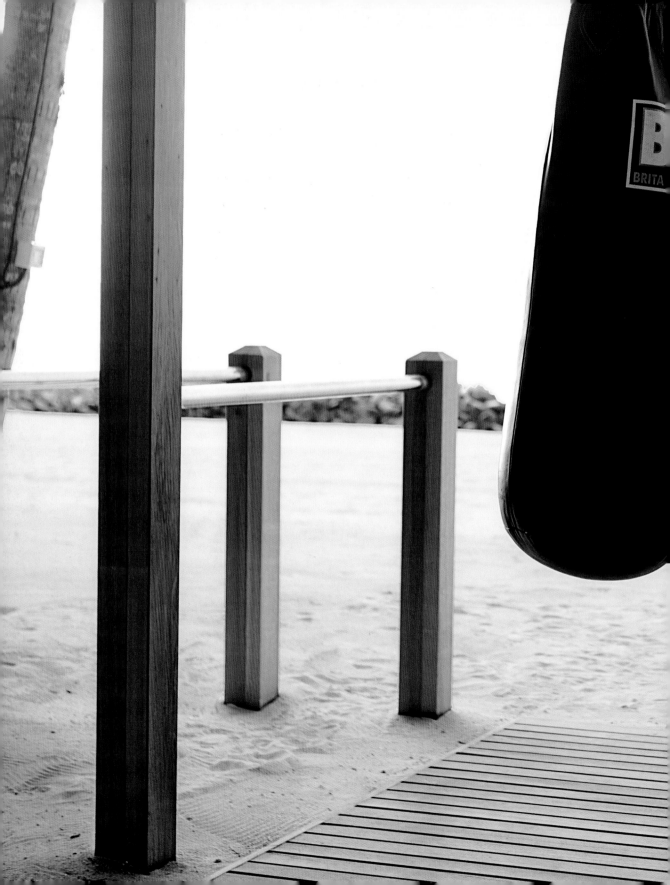

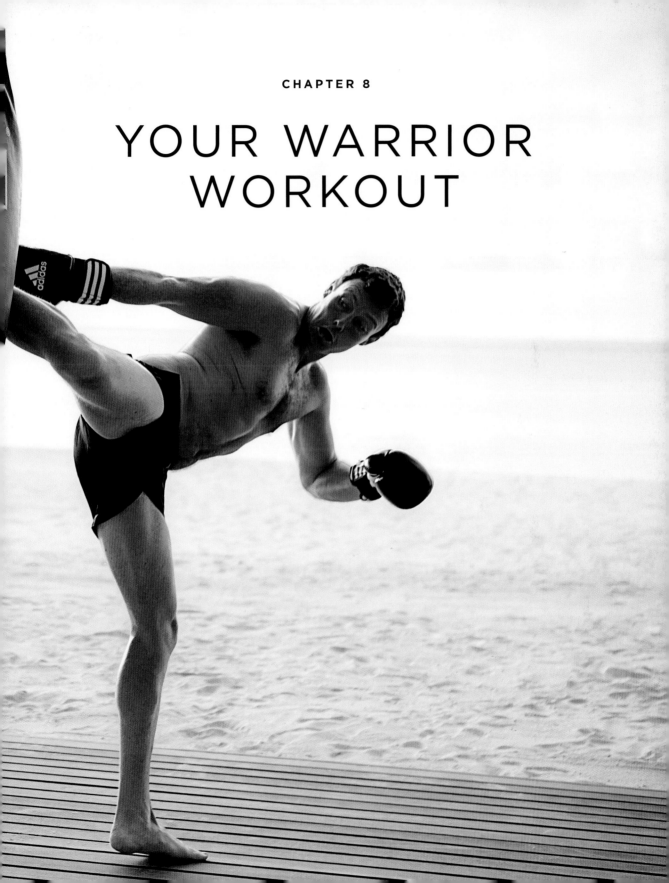

CHAPTER 8

YOUR WARRIOR WORKOUT

TIME TO WORK OUT

I want you to succeed and get as much benefit as possible from all the movement programmes that follow. They have have all been designed to strengthen you, strip fat, improve your posture and increase your athletic ability. These movements are the basis for everything I do. I use these exercises to stay strong, fast and lean. I can do them anywhere in the world and the only equipment I need is whatever I can find lying around wherever I am at the time. Use the programmes to build a strong foundation and test yourself. Find out what your body can do.

One of the best things you can do is find a training partner as they will keep you motivated and accountable. Having a buddy also makes the process more fun and a healthy sense of competition is a great way to stay on track when you might otherwise falter or compromise. My best friend is a gentleman by the name of Justin Alexander and we have been kicking and punching and training with each other since we were thirteen years old. The guy is a fierce competitor and never gives up, which motivates me to train harder and be better. We both love boxing and Brazilian jiu jitsu and so for over twenty years we have been learning from whoever we can and testing each other's will and skill. This has kept me focused and made me stronger every day.

I have also had the huge honour of learning Brazilian jiu jitsu from perhaps the greatest champ of all time, Roger Gracie. He has taught me that you can be the best in the world and still remain humble and willing to learn every day. I also once had the privilege of training with and learning from Georges St. Pierre, one of the best pound-for-pound fighters on the planet. He is the strongest human being I have ever encountered and is one of the best examples of what the human body is capable of. The one thing all these guys have in common is that they never give up and will always find a way rather than looking for an excuse. So get busy, start moving and get it done!

*top tip
If you don't have a log to hand, a water bottle, a dumb bell, barbell, cricket bat etc, will also do nicely

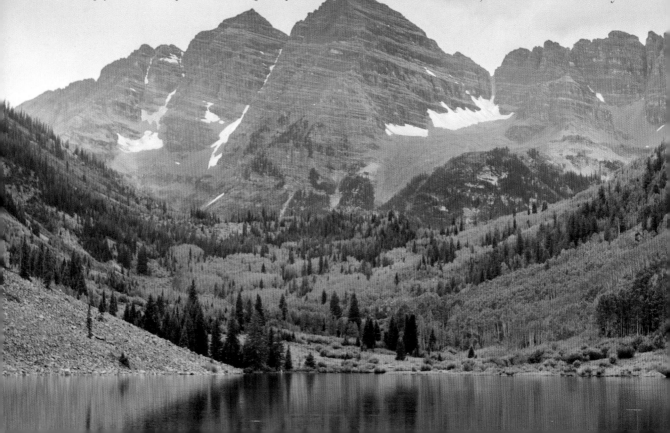

UPPER BODY WARRIOR WORKOUT

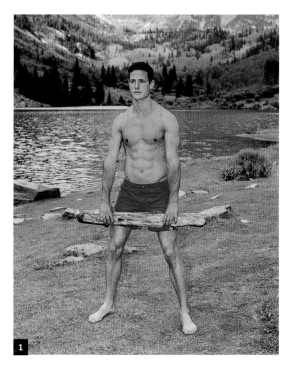

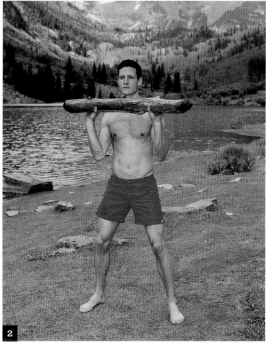

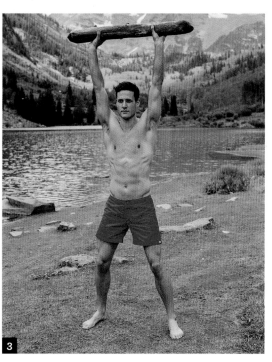

Reverse grip bicep curl to shoulder press

Start position:
1. Stand tall with your feet slightly wider than shoulder width apart. Hold the log by your thighs with an overhand grip and hands shoulder width apart.

The movement:
2. Bend at the elbows and curl the log up to level with your shoulders while keeping your wrists locked.
3. Keeping your core set, extend your arms so that the log is held above your head.
4. Slowly, bend your elbows and lower the log in front of your chest, then straighten your arms until the log returns to the start position.
Repeat 15 times.

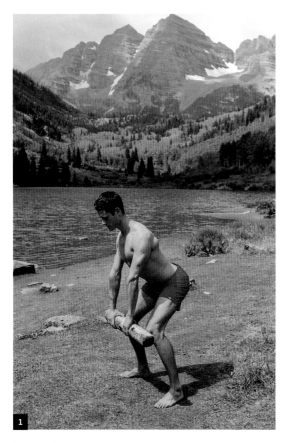

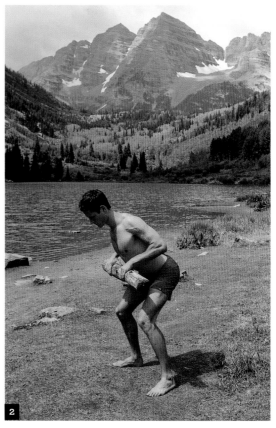

Bent over row reverse grip

Start position:

1. Hold the log with an overhand grip, hands about shoulder-width apart at arm's length. Bend at your hips and knees, until your torso is at a 30° angle, whilst maintaining a straight back.

The movement:

2. While keeping your core engaged, pull the log up towards your belly button. Squeeze your shoulder blades together and keep your wrists locked. Slowly lower the log back to the start position.

Repeat 12 times.

*top tip
There is no such thing as failure, only feedback. You will get there if you keep trying and it will be worth it.

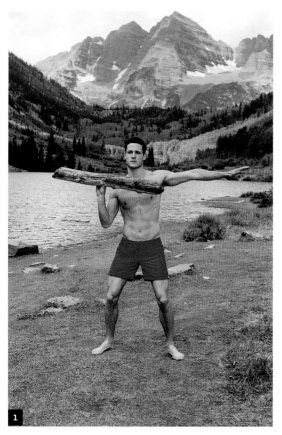

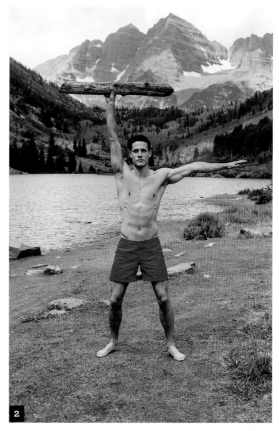

Single arm shoulder press

Start position:

1. Stand tall with your feet slightly wider than shoulder width apart. Maintain perfect posture (straight back, chest up, ears over shoulders). Grip the log (underhand grip) with your right hand and hold the log level with your right shoulder.

The movement:

2. Set your core and straighten your right arm above your head until your left arm is fully extended whilst maintaining perfect posture and a fixed wrist.

3. Slowly, bend at the elbow and lower the log back to the starting position.

Repeat this 12 times and then switch to the left arm and perform 12 repetitions.

*top tip

When you engage your core, draw your belly gently towards your spine – not a full, harsh suck-in, just a gentle pull.

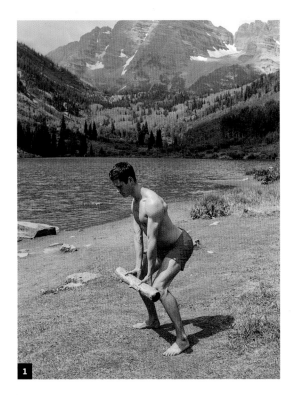

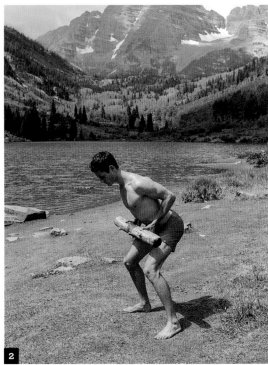

Bent over row
underhand grip

Start position:

1. Hold the log with an underhand grip, hands about shoulder-width apart at arm's length. Bend at your hips and knees, until your torso is 30° above parallel to the floor whilst maintaining a straight back.

The movement:

2. While keeping your core engaged, pull the log up towards your belly button. Squeeze your shoulder blades together and keep your wrists locked. Slowly lower the log back to the start position.

Repeat 12 times.

*top tip

Remember why you're doing this.
The results will be amazing.

LOWER BODY WARRIOR WORKOUT

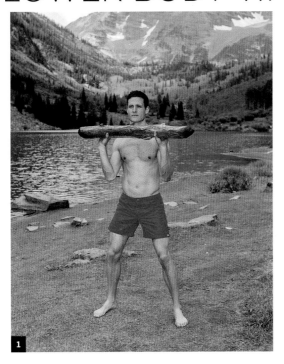

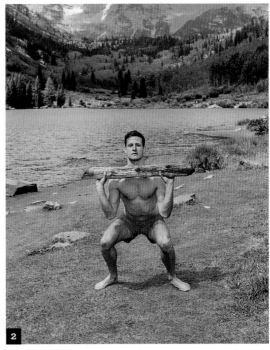

Squat press

Start position:
1. Stand with your feet slightly wider than shoulder width apart with an overhand grip of the log. Start with the log in front of your chin, level with your shoulders.

The movement:
2. Keeping your heels on the ground, bend your knees and sit your hips back and stick your butt out. Squat until your thighs are at least parallel with the floor, while maintaining perfect posture (straight back, chest up, ears over shoulders).
3. As you push up through your heels to return to a standing position, fully extend your arms above your head.
4. Once completed, slowly bend at your elbows and return the log back down to the starting position.
Repeat 15 times.

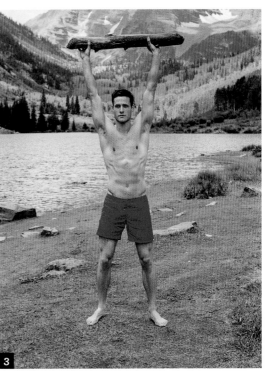

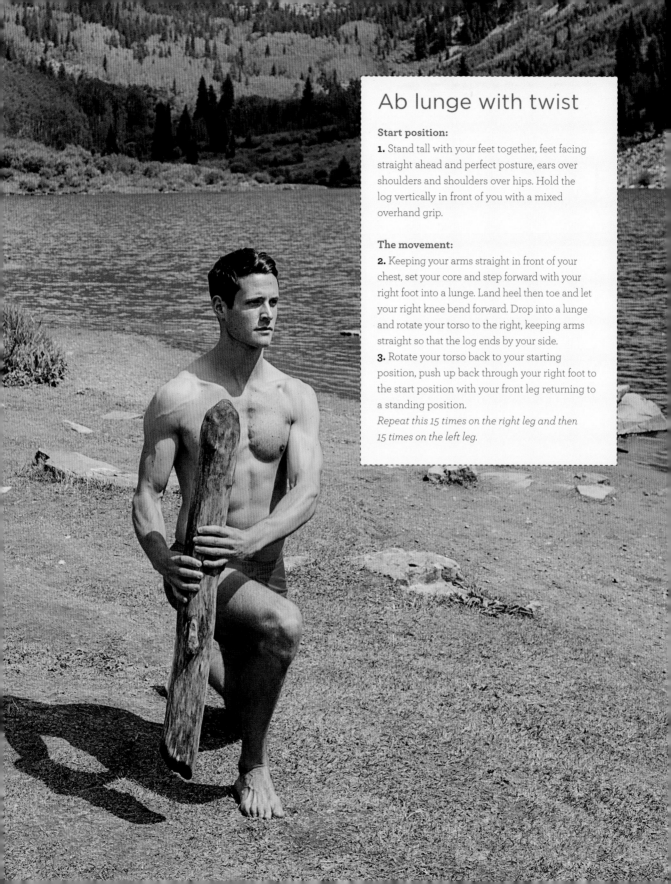

Ab lunge with twist

Start position:
1. Stand tall with your feet together, feet facing straight ahead and perfect posture, ears over shoulders and shoulders over hips. Hold the log vertically in front of you with a mixed overhand grip.

The movement:
2. Keeping your arms straight in front of your chest, set your core and step forward with your right foot into a lunge. Land heel then toe and let your right knee bend forward. Drop into a lunge and rotate your torso to the right, keeping arms straight so that the log ends by your side.
3. Rotate your torso back to your starting position, push up back through your right foot to the start position with your front leg returning to a standing position.
Repeat this 15 times on the right leg and then 15 times on the left leg.

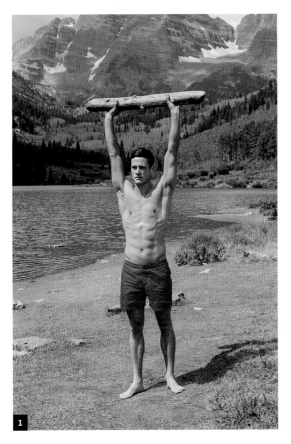

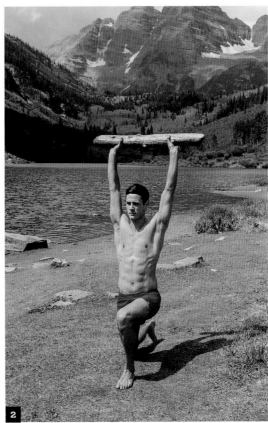

Overhead lunge

Start position:

1. Stand tall with your feet together, feet facing straight ahead and perfect posture – ears over shoulders and shoulders over hips. Hold the log straight above your head with arms fully extended and an overhand grip on the log.

The movement:

2. Set your core muscles and step forward into a lunge with your arms staying straight above your head. Land heel then toe and let your front knee bend forward.

3. Push up back to the start position with your front leg returning to a standing position.

Repeat this 15 times on the right leg and then 15 times on the left leg.

*top tip

Always remember, your body loves to move. Cherish it, express your joy, run fast, jump high!

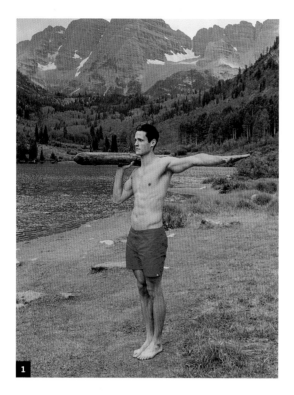

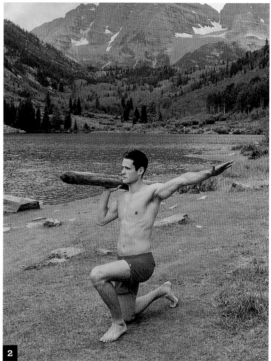

Lunge get up with log

Start position:

1. Stand tall with your feet together, feet facing straight ahead and perfect posture – ears over shoulders and shoulders over hips. Hold the log with an overhand grip with the log resting on your right shoulder.

The movement:

2. Set your core and step backwards with your right foot into a reverse lunge while maintaining the log resting on your shoulder. Land onto your right toe, bending at your left knee.

3. Slowly, let your right knee rest onto the floor then bring your left foot back to end in a tall kneeling position.

4. From here, bring your right foot forward and step up so that you end standing in perfect posture.

Repeat this for 10 repetitions with the right leg and then 10 times with the left leg.

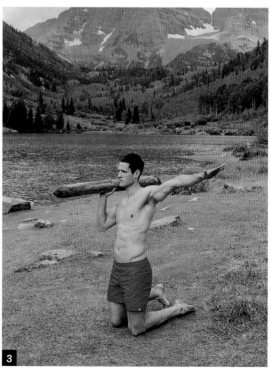

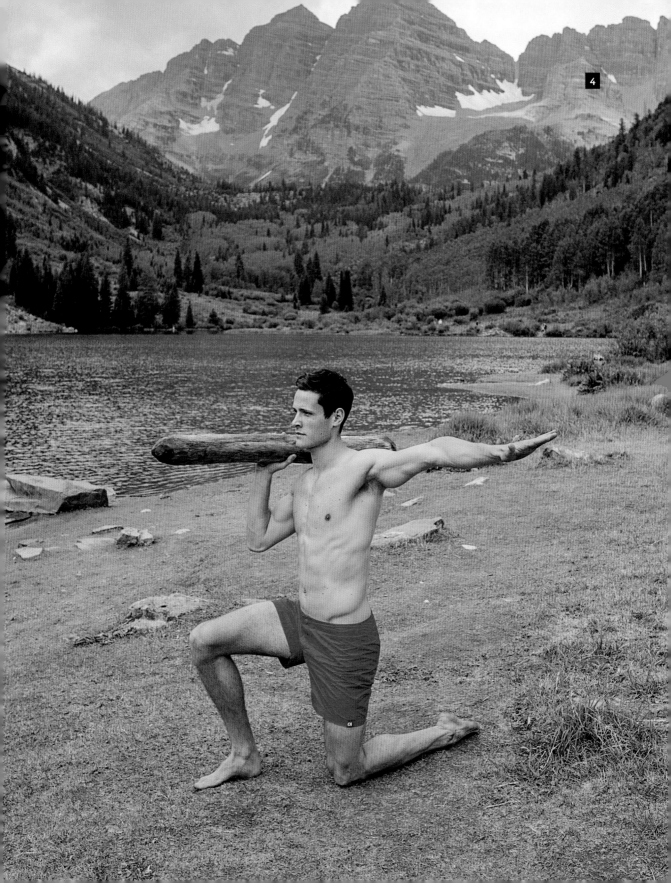

THE WARRIOR AB WORKOUT

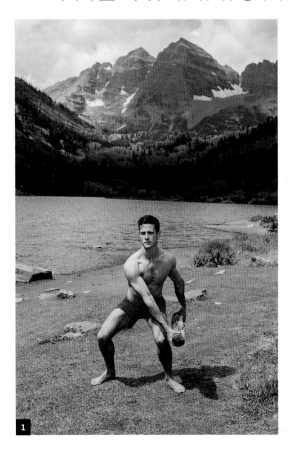

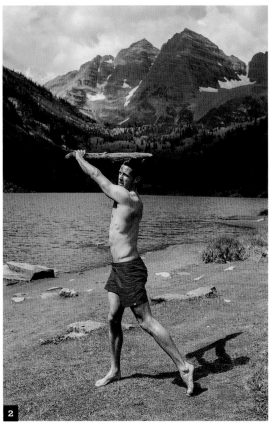

Wood chop

Start position:

Stand tall with your feet slightly wider than shoulder width apart. Hold the log to the side of your left hip with a mixed grip, hands shoulder width apart.

The movement:

1. Squat until your thighs are at least parallel with the floor, while maintaining perfect posture (straight back, chest up, ears over shoulders).

2. As you push up through your heels to return to a standing position, lift the log diagonally across your body until your arms are fully extended. Once completed, return the log back to the start position.

Perform 10 repetitions from right to left, then 10 repetitions from left to right

*top tip
Using weights accelerates the fat-burning process.

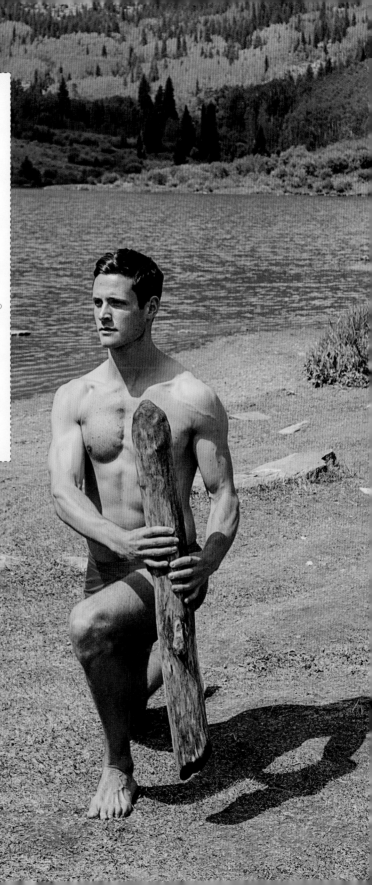

Ab Lunge with Twist

Start position:
1. Stand tall with your feet together, feet facing straight ahead and perfect posture, ears over shoulders and shoulders over hips. Hold the log vertically in front of you with a mixed overhand grip.

The movement:
2. Keeping your arms straight in front of your chest, set your core and step forward with your left foot into a lunge. Land heel then toe and let your left knee bend forward. Drop into a lunge and rotate your torso to the left, keeping arms straight so that the log ends by your side.
3. Rotate your torso back to your starting position, push up back through your left foot to the start position with your front leg returning to a standing position.
Repeat this 15 times on the left leg and then 15 times on the right leg.

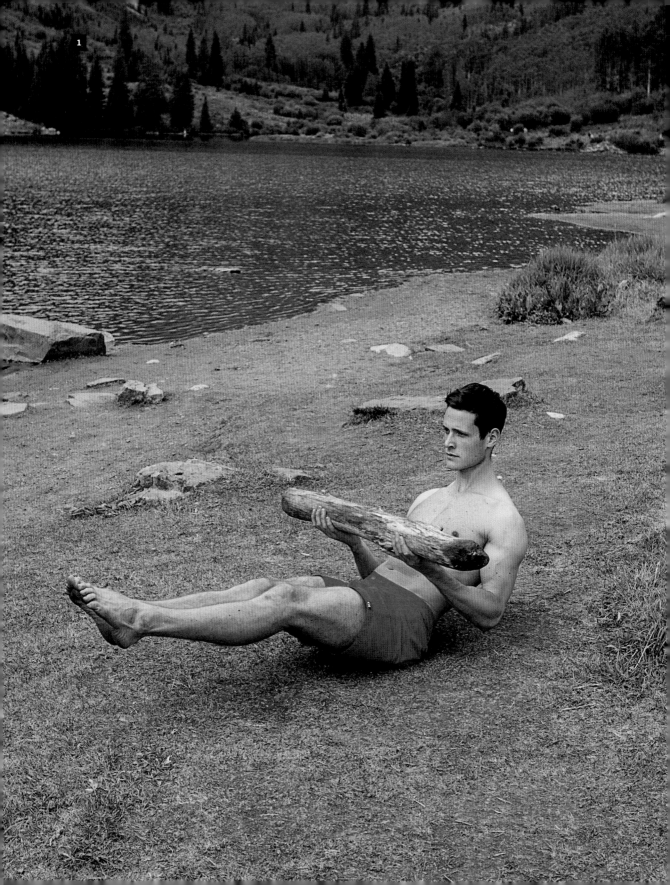

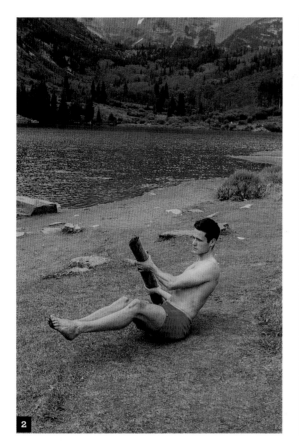

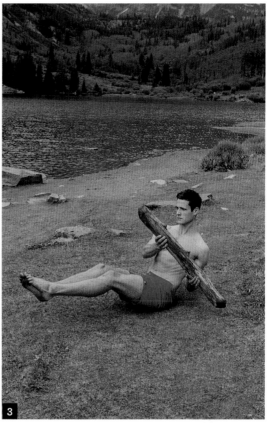

Kayak sit up

Start position:

1. Begin seated on the floor with knees slightly bent. Grip the log with an underhand grip and hands shoulder-width apart. Keep your elbows bent. Find your balance and raise your feet off the floor so that you are balancing on your buttocks.

The movement:

2. While keeping your elbows bent and chest up, slowly turn your torso to the right so that the log is by your right side.

3. Twist to the left so that the log is by your left side. Keep your elbows bent and chest up for the whole set. *Continue this for 40 twists, alternating from right to left.*

*top tip

Work with your body, not against it. Listen to what it is telling you.

20-MINUTE WARRIOR BLAST WITH CARDIO WORKOUT

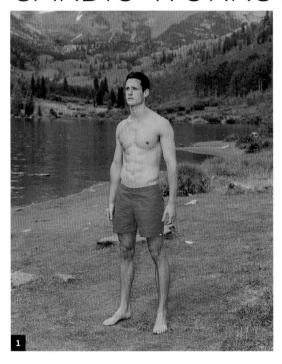

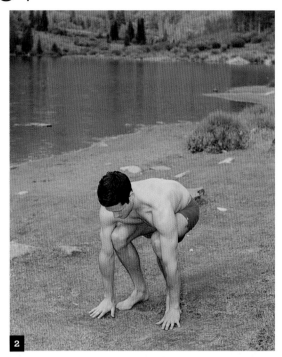

Burpee

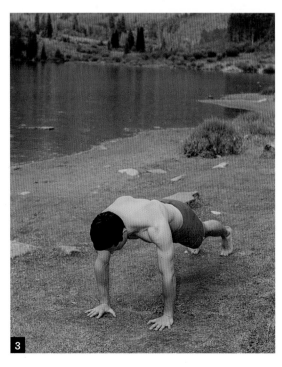

Start position:
1. Begin standing in an upright position with feet shoulder width apart and with perfect posture.

The movement:
2. Bend at the knees and hips and go as low to the ground as possible whilst keeping your back straight, and chest up. Place both hands on the floor.
3. Jump both feet back together so that you end in a push up position, keeping your abdominals engaged. Jump both feet back so that you return to the crouched position with your head and chest up.
4. From this crouched position, jump up into the air and land softly with knees slightly bent.
Repeat the whole movement continuously for 30 seconds.

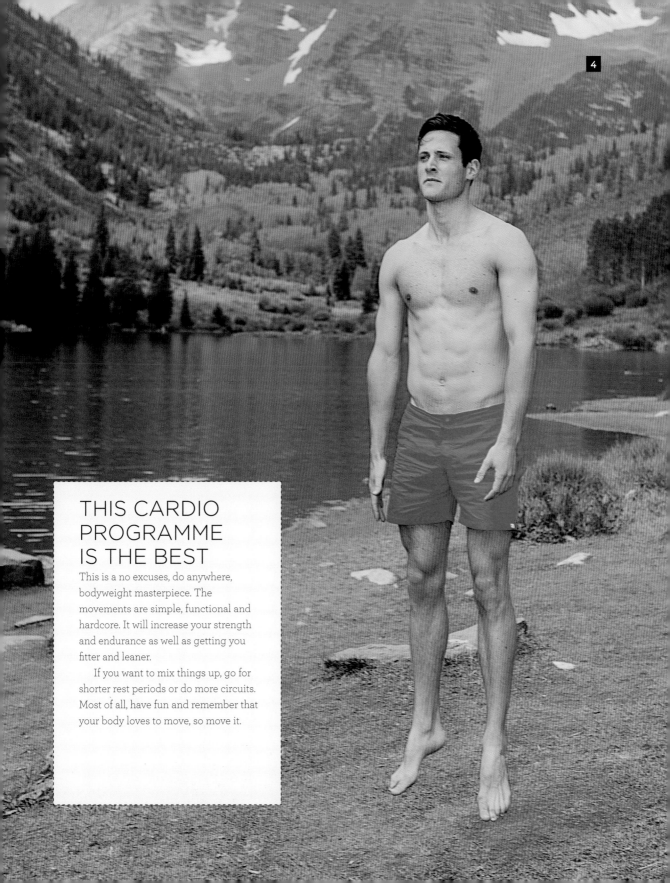

THIS CARDIO PROGRAMME IS THE BEST

This is a no excuses, do anywhere, bodyweight masterpiece. The movements are simple, functional and hardcore. It will increase your strength and endurance as well as getting you fitter and leaner.

If you want to mix things up, go for shorter rest periods or do more circuits. Most of all, have fun and remember that your body loves to move, so move it.

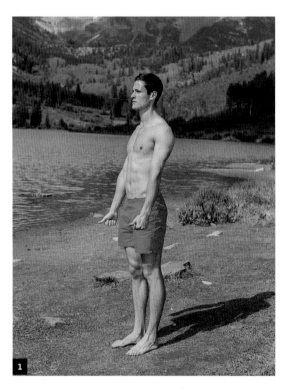

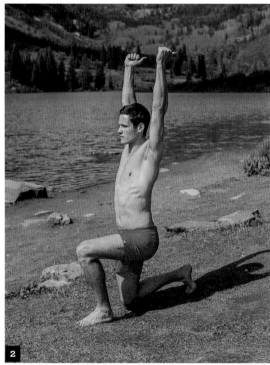

Disco lunge

Start position:

1. Begin standing in an upright position with feet together and perfect posture. Begin with both arms by your side with hands clenched and thumbs up.

The movement:

2. Set your core and step forward into a lunge. As you lunge forward with your left foot, extend both arms above your head to make a Y shape. Land heel then toe and let your front knee bend forward.

3. Push up back to the start position, returning with your front leg to a standing position and your arms to the side. *Repeat this for 30 seconds.*

*top tip

This is my 10-second rule to good posture: stand up straight, keep your back straight with your ears over your shoulders and your shoulders over your hips. Look straight ahead and think tall, right through your spine and through the top of your head.

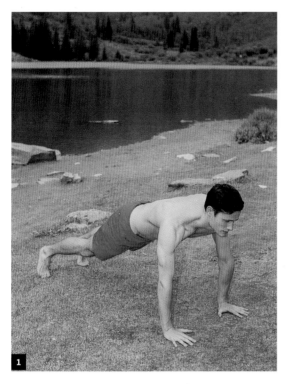

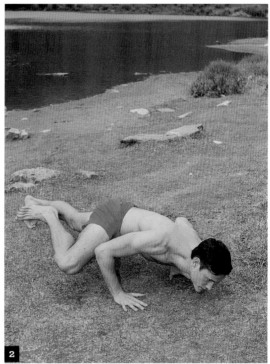

Spiderman push up

Start position:
Start in a push up position, hands directly under shoulders, abs engaged, neck in line with spine.

The movement:
1. As you lower your body towards the floor slowly, lift your right foot off the floor and drive your right knee high towards your right elbow.
2. Then reverse the movement with your leg and push your body back up to the starting position. Then repeat this but with the opposite knee.
Keep alternating knees for 30 seconds.

*top tip
Don't waste time with guilt – keep going and do your best.

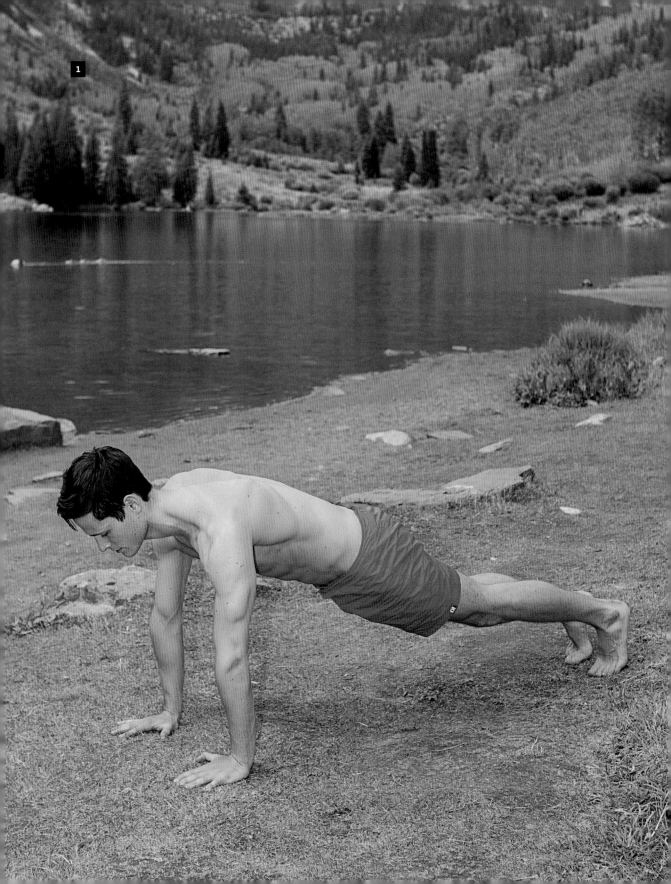

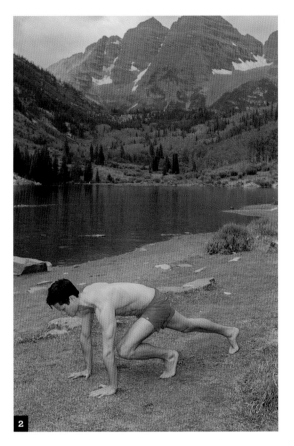

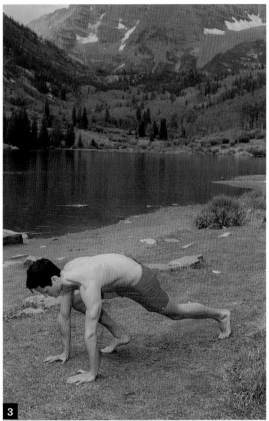

Mountain climber

Start position:

1. Start in a push up position, hands directly under shoulders, abs engaged, neck in line with spine.

The movement:

2. Keeping your hips square to the floor, drive your right knee up towards your chest and extend your left leg back.

3. Keep your abs engaged the whole time as both feet switch positions. Don't let the foot of the knee you drive up towards your chest touch the floor.

Continue this for 30 seconds.

*top tip

Check your starting position. Make sure your hands are directly under your shoulders, abs engaged, neck in line with your spine.

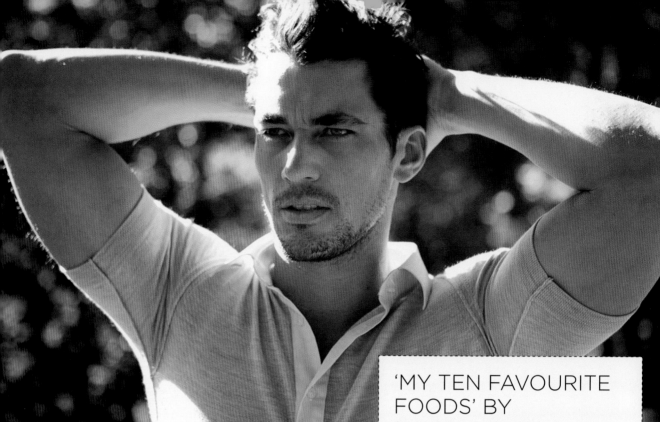

GET DAVID GANDY'S BODY

David Gandy's body is proof that living Clean & Lean really works. His athletic body is the envy of many men... and women. (The other thing about David is, he's a really good person, a decent and highly principled man who cares deeply about people. We like him a lot.)

He started training at Bodyism with Nathalie four years ago in order to train for the Dolce and Gabbana Light Blue 2 shoot and filming. It was an entirely unique approach to training and nutrition, something completely different for his mind and body and a programme designed for a healthy body and a happy life. His sessions involved Bodyism circuit training, similar to the workout that follows here, and interval training. He also followed a Clean & Lean nutrition programme. The results speak for themselves and when David needs a super lean, cut physique, there is only one programme he turns to.

'MY TEN FAVOURITE FOODS' BY DAVID GANDY

David loves food, like the rest of us, but he is intelligent about what he eats and when he has his cheat meals. These are the top ten foods that David eats when he wants to get into top shape. They all help him to decrease his fat %, increase muscle mass and stay healthy and energetic.

1. Eggs: packed with vitamins, minerals, good fats and protein

2. Alaskan Salmon: high quality protein and Omega-3

3. Chicken: a lean source of protein

4. Almonds: healthy fats, vitamin E, iron and magnesium

5. Avocado: healthy fat and fibre

6. Spinach: packed with iron, antioxidants and vitamins

7. Sweet potato: a healthy carbohydrate and packed with vitamins and antioxidants

8. Broccoli: full of folate, iron and vitamin K

9. Raspberries: vitamin C and antioxidants

10. Coconut oil: the ideal oil to use for all types of cooking. Increases thyroid activity and speeds up the metabolism

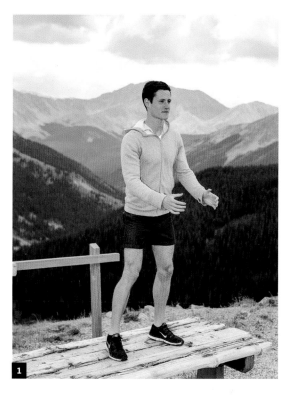

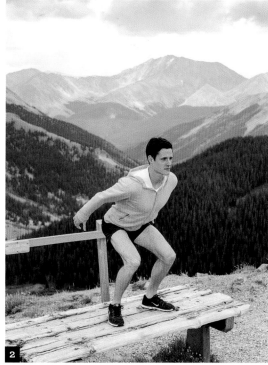

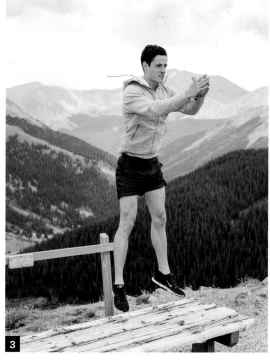

1. Jumping squats

Start position:
1. Stand with your feet hip width apart.

The movement:
2. Sit back in to a squat with your weight on your heels. Bring your elbows back and, when you start to jump up, the arm force will help you jump higher.
3. Extend your knees and hips and then land softly onto bent knees again.
Repeat 15 times.

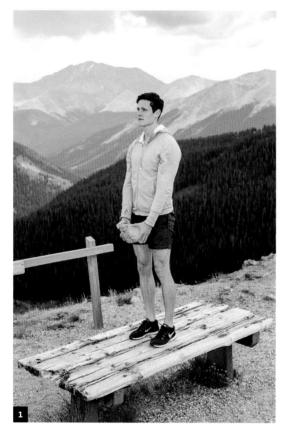

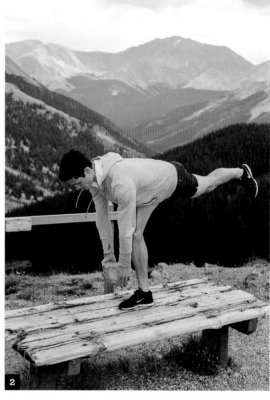

2. Single leg Romanian dead lifts

Start position:

1. Stand holding a weight in both hands.

The movement:

2. Hinge over at your waist. Bring your left leg up behind you and aim to reach your hands to your standing foot.

Repeat 10 times on each leg.

*top tip

Return to the starting position by switching on your glutes (your gluteus maximus, the main muscles in your bottom).

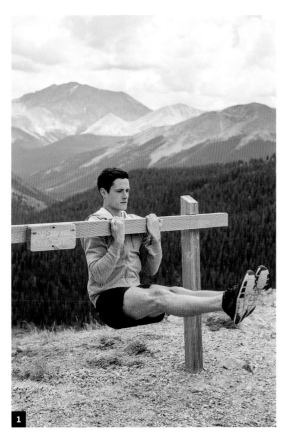

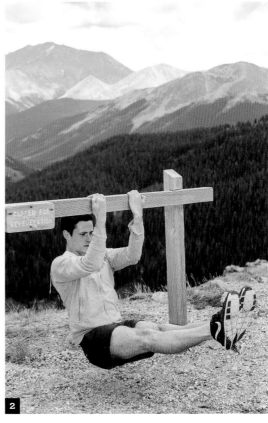

3. Chin ups

Start position:
1. If you have access to one (in your local gym or park, for example), pull yourself up on a chin up bar.

The movement:
2. Lower yourself down as slowly as possible and hold the position for 20–40 seconds.
Repeat 3 times.

*top tip

This isometric exercise is great but it's tough. If you want to make it easier, do more reps (without holding the position) and, when you're ready, step it up by holding for a few seconds.

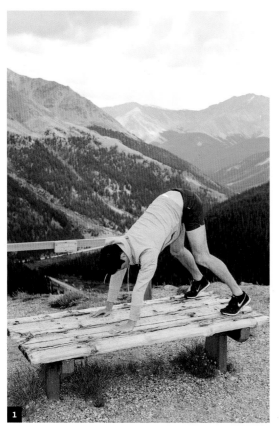

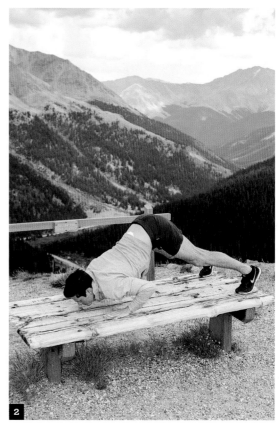

4. Flowing push up

Start position:

1. Get into the downward facing dog position, a popular yoga move.

The movement:

2. Bend your arms and lower your chest towards the ground.

3. Just before you reach the floor, straighten out your arms and arch your back and look up towards the ceiling. Go back to the starting position.

Repeat 10 times, or until your perfect technique is lost.

*top tip

In downward dog, keep your knees slightly bent and your heels lifted away from the floor. Stretch and lengthen your back. Breathe out and stretch your heels onto (or towards) the floor. Straighten your knees but don't 'lock them'. Keep your fingers pressed firmly into the floor and firm your shoulder blades against your back. Keep your head between your upper arms but don't let it hang.

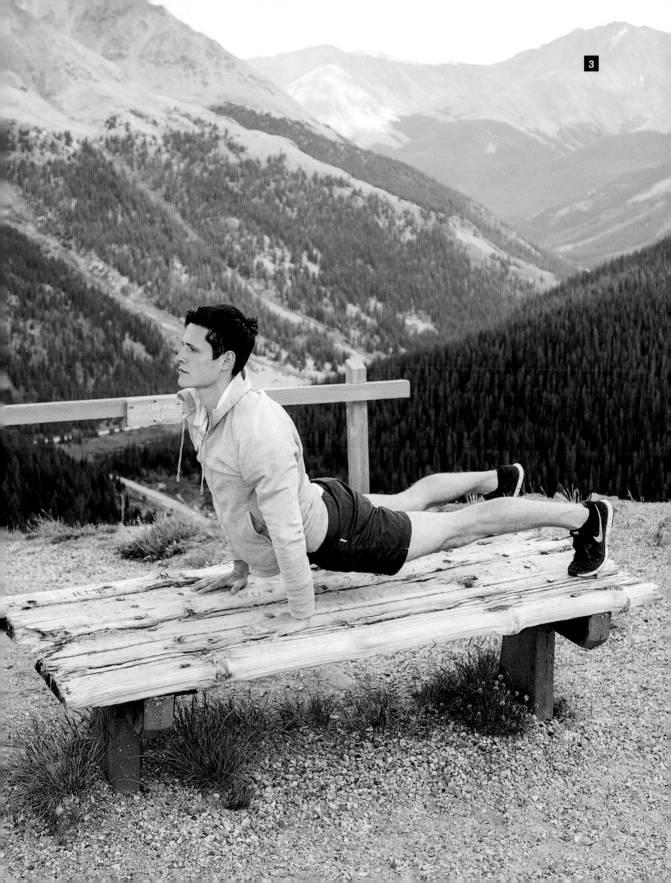

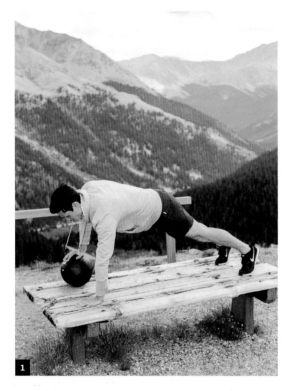

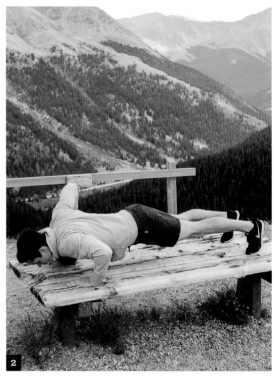

5. Push up with one hand on a medicine ball

Start position:

1. Get into a push up position with one hand on a medicine ball.

The movement:

2. Keep your tummy tight and lower your body towards the floor.

3. Drive your body up away from the floor and the ball quickly and land with the other hand on the ball.

Do as many as you can – 14 ideally.

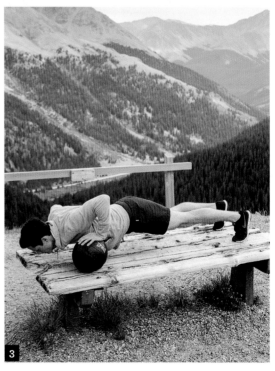

*top tip
This is incredibly hard so if you can't manage it, start with straightforward push ups instead.

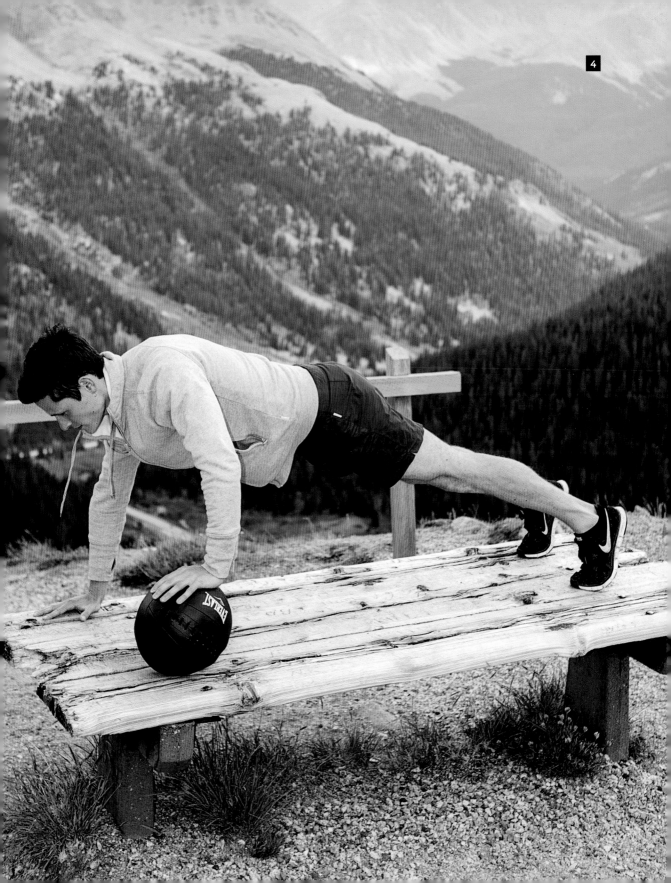

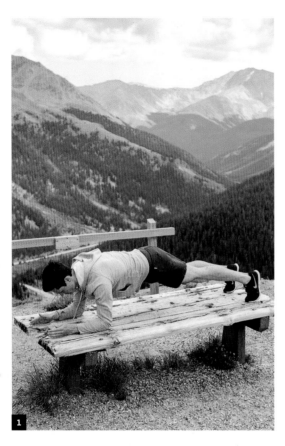

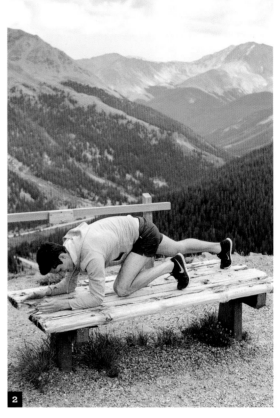

4

6. Plank with single leg knee tucks

Start position:

1. Get into a plank position by lying face down on the floor and raise yourself into a push-up-style position, with your forearms, elbows and tips of your toes supporting you. Keep your stomach muscles tight and your hips up so your body forms a straight line from your head to your feet.

The movement:

2. First, slowly bring your right knee towards your chest, second, bring the right knee in towards the outside of the right triceps and third, bring the right knee in towards the left triceps. Repeat with the other leg.

Repeat 15 times on each leg.

*top tip
You can also use a Swiss exercise ball if you have one to hand. They are good as they help stabilise and engage the core muscles.

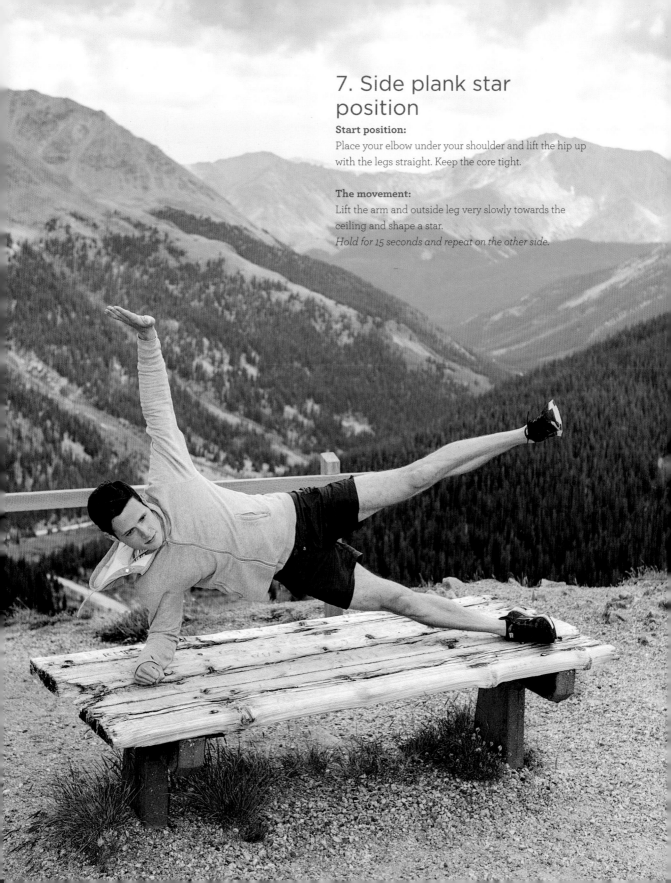

7. Side plank star position

Start position:
Place your elbow under your shoulder and lift the hip up with the legs straight. Keep the core tight.

The movement:
Lift the arm and outside leg very slowly towards the ceiling and shape a star.
Hold for 15 seconds and repeat on the other side.

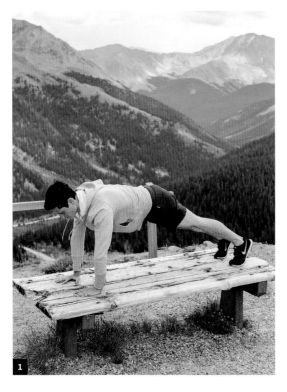

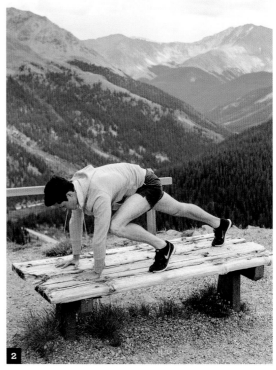

8. Mountain climbers

Start position:

1. Get into a plank position.

The movement:

2. Bring one knee at a time into the chest, very quickly.

3. It should take about 1 second to change the legs around.
Continue this for 30 seconds.

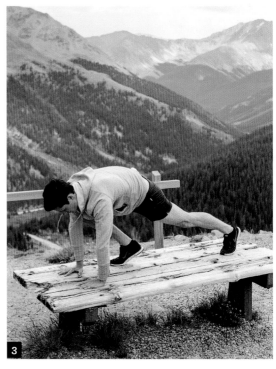

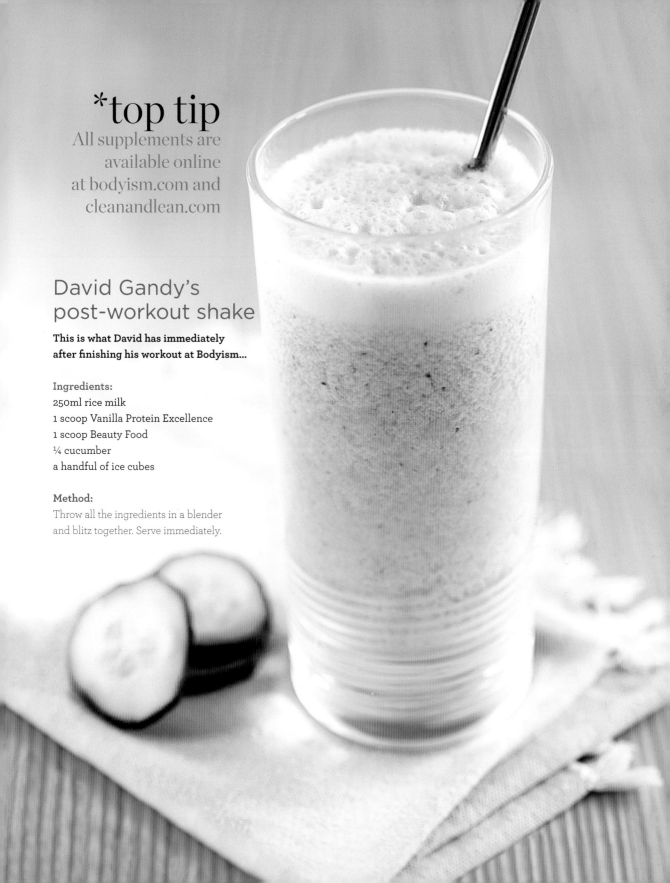

David Gandy's post-workout shake

This is what David has immediately after finishing his workout at Bodyism...

Ingredients:
250ml rice milk
1 scoop Vanilla Protein Excellence
1 scoop Beauty Food
¼ cucumber
a handful of ice cubes

Method:
Throw all the ingredients in a blender and blitz together. Serve immediately.

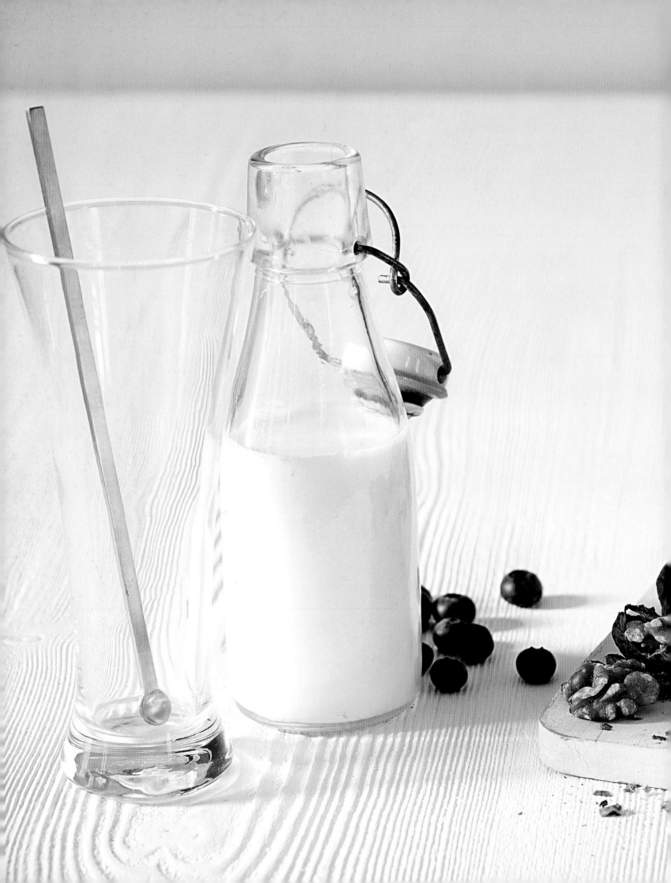

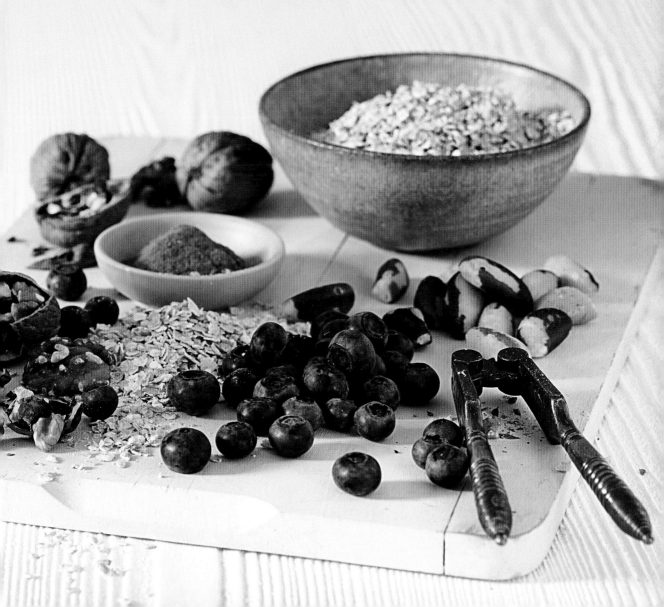

CHAPTER 9

EASY MEALS
FOR MEN

This chapter includes all my favourite Clean & Lean recipes. Because my clients are busy people who often travel a lot or work in offices, all the meals in this chapter are unfussy, quick and easy to make. As a general rule, all your meals should include a hefty portion of protein (at least the size of your palm – not a scrappy bit of chicken tucked into a pre-packaged, shop-bought sandwich), a handful of something green (like broccoli, courgette, salad etc), something colourful (like pepper, or some bright berries to finish) and some good fat (like nuts, hummus, a drizzle of oil or some avocado).

BREAKFAST

Most of us start the day with the entirely wrong breakfast. We often tend to wait to have it until we get to work, meaning more than an hour passes between waking up and eating. Plus, most of us have breakfasts made up almost entirely of carbs, like toast or cereal. If you get your breakfast wrong, you'll feel tired and hungry throughout the day. But if you get it right, your body will become a fat-fighting, energised machine all day long. Here's how to get it right.

✳ Protein should always be a major part of your breakfast. You need protein – found in eggs, meat, fish or dairy – to build muscle and keep you full. Never have a carbs-only (or mainly carb) breakfast. The same goes for a sugary breakfast – so avoid cereal and croissants.

✳ Have a little fat. Found in nuts, avocado, oily fish and olive oil, good, healthy fat helps to keep you alert and energised. The man-boosting mix of protein and fat also slows the absorption of carbohydrates into your bloodstream which keeps your blood-sugar levels (and therefore your energy levels) steady. A carbs-only breakfast has the opposite effect and will leave you hungry and tired by mid-morning.

✳ As well as protein and fat, eat something green at breakfast. Whether it's cold salad or fruit (half a sliced avocado, an apple, some cucumber, etc.), cooked vegetables (I've been known to have broccoli for breakfast – sounds weird, but it makes me feel amazing all day) or a smoothie with something green in it (kale, cabbage, apples, etc.) I strongly advise you to get a hit of vitamins first thing.

✳ Eat within an hour of waking up. Even if you're not hungry, eating soon after waking speeds up your metabolism, which makes fat burning easier. Why? Because if you leave it any longer, your body thinks you're starving it (remember, it's been around ten hours since your last meal), so it clings on to calories.

✳ Take Body Brilliance every morning – a fat-burning blend of antioxidants. I have this every day and I recommend it to my clients too. Just mix one scoop with water and drink it alongside your breakfast. Available at www.bodyism.com.

✳ Drink a cup of cooled boiled water with a slice of lemon in it when you first wake up. It cleans out your system, hydrating you and improving your digestion. Other good options include green tea or just a glass of water. Have one of these before your coffee or tea, which should only be drunk after you've eaten breakfast. When you do drink tea or coffee, keep it as Clean & Lean as possible. That means organic milk, no sugar and the best-quality tea or coffee you can afford.

✳ Remember: leftovers aren't just for lunch. I often eat whatever's in the fridge from the night before for breakfast. That could be some cold cooked chicken and broccoli. It may sound weird, but it's better for you than processed, sugary cereal or toast. Add a handful of nuts and you have the perfect mix of protein, fat and greens.

AFTER 8PM

Don't eat between 8pm and 8am (or thereabouts). A recent study from the Salk Institute in California found that our bodies are hardwired to expect a twelve-hour fast overnight. This, say the scientists, is how our ancestors lived and it enables our livers to burn fat efficiently overnight. However, the relatively recent phenomenon of eating dinner later – or worse, post-dinner snacking right up until bedtime – means that most of us are failing to fast for twelve hours. So not eating between 8pm and 8am also works on another level: if you don't eat anything between dinner and breakfast you'll cut out all those unnecessary junk snacks.

DON'T SKIP LUNCH

When my clients first come to see me, they often explain that they start the day with good intentions and a good breakfast, but that it's all gone wrong by lunchtime. Because they're so busy with work they either skip lunch or grab something fast, carb-heavy and processed. They eat it quickly at their desk so they can get back to work and then wonder why they feel bloated, tired and uncomfortable all afternoon.

Most popular 'desk lunches' contain barely any protein, which is vital for keeping you full. So always eat protein at lunch (at least a palm-sized amount – a scrappy bit of chicken in a sandwich doesn't count as it'll leave you feeling hungry again very soon), along with some good fat (e.g. half an avocado, a small handful or nuts and seeds, or a good drizzle of olive oil) and something green (e.g. lettuce, cucumber or broccoli) and, ideally, something brightly coloured (tomatoes, peppers, berries, etc.).

Take at least a 20 minute break for your lunch and really savour it. Otherwise, you 'stress eat', you don't chew thoroughly and your body won't absorb the nutrients efficiently. Concentrate on your food, not your work, so your body registers you are eating and signals you are full.

Another good tip is to eat leftovers for lunch. Whatever I cook for dinner, I often have cold the next day for lunch with a good handful of salad or vegetables. This is especially good for men who work in offices and can't cook lunch.

CLEAN & LEAN DINNERS

In theory, you have more time to prepare and eat dinner than you do breakfast or lunch – especially if you work in an office and rush out the door at breakfast time and eat lunch at your desk. However, dinner is also a time when you're likely to be exhausted from your day and tempted to eat something quick and processed. That's why some of the recipes here take less than ten minutes to make. Others take a little longer, so they're probably better for a weekend dinner. If you make sure you always have certain foods in your kitchen – protein (chicken, fish, eggs, a pot of homemade hummus, etc.) and lots of vegetables (especially green ones), you'll be able to make something quickly that will help calm you down and unwind before bed.

As with breakfast and lunch, it's important to have a good serving of protein with dinner. This will keep you full (and away from post-dinner snacks) and feed your muscles. Avoid sugar and caffeine because they're stimulants that disrupt sleep. Avoid alcohol, too – despite what most people think about alcohol calming them down in the evenings and helping them get to sleep, alcohol is actually a stimulant that will reduce the quality of your sleep. It's also full of sugar, which will stimulate you further. If you must have a drink in the evenings – and it's a good idea to have several alcohol-free days a week – have a small glass of red wine or a vodka with a squeeze of lemon or lime. Red wine contains a small number of health-boosting antioxidants (but don't kid yourself it's healthy, it's just less bad for you than a large glass of sugary white wine) and the vodka is a pretty clean option compared to a sugary beer.

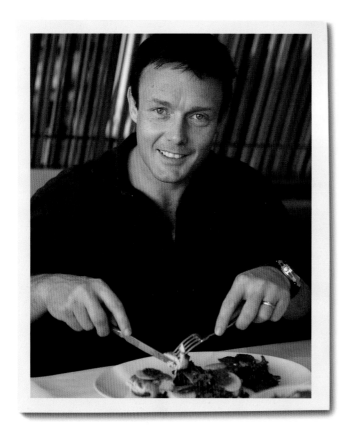

JAMES' FAVOURITE BREAKFAST
Haddock, Eggs and Asparagus on Rye
Serves 1

1 x 200g fillet undyed smoked haddock
2 organic eggs
70g asparagus
2 slices rye bread, toasted if you like
sea salt and freshly ground black pepper

Method
1. Heat a medium frying pan of water until boiling. Add the haddock fillet, cover with a lid then turn off the heat and leave for 5 minutes.

2. Poach the eggs in a separate pan in simmering water for about 4 minutes or until the whites are set but the yolks are still soft. Steam the asparagus at the same time.

3. To serve, divide the haddock between the rye bread slices. Top each with a poached egg and asparagus spears and season to taste.

*top tip
This is what I eat on a training day as the rye bread is great for an extra burst of energy.

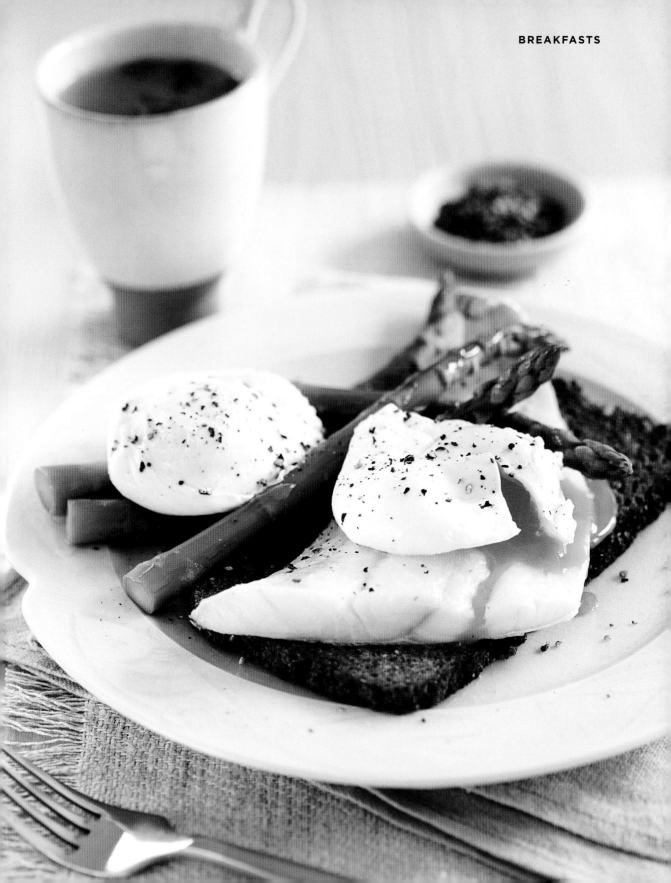

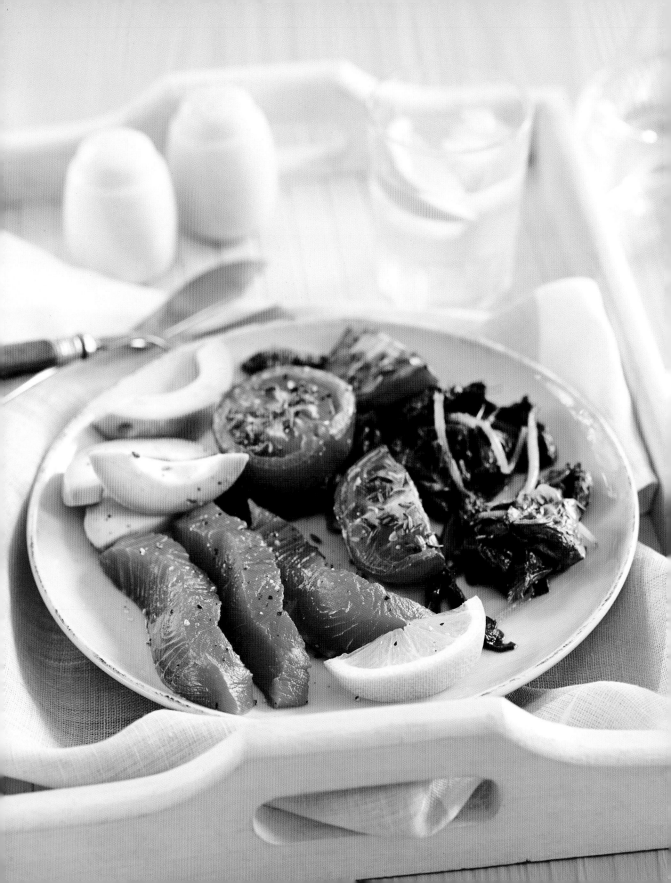

Super Clean & Lean Breakfast

Serves 2

3 small plum tomatoes
2 tablespoons extra-virgin olive oil
sea salt and freshly ground black pepper
1½ teaspoons cumin seeds
500g spinach, trimmed and chopped
4–6 x 50g pieces salmon sashimi
1 avocado, peeled and sliced
½ lemon

Method

1. Preheat the oven to 200°C/400°F/gas mark 6.

2. Cut the tomatoes in half and place on a baking tray. Drizzle with 1 tablespoon olive oil, sprinkle with salt and pepper and scatter the cumin seeds on top. Roast for about 15–20 minutes. (These can be cooked up to a day ahead and served cold, or reheated in a hot oven for 5 minutes.)

3. Heat the remaining olive oil in a large frying pan over a low heat. Add the spinach, cover and cook for 5 minutes, stirring occasionally until wilted. Season well, cover again and cook for another 5 minutes, then remove from the heat.

4. Arrange everything on 2 plates. Add a squeeze of lemon and serve immediately.

James' Fish Hash: White Fish, Sweet Potato and Onions Sautéed in Coconut Oil

Serves 2

500ml water
2 cloves garlic, unpeeled, left whole
1 small white onion, unpeeled, left whole
sea salt and freshly ground black pepper
400g firm-fleshed white fish fillets, cut into 10cm chunks
1 tablespoon coconut oil
1 small white onion, peeled and finely chopped
1 sweet potato, peeled and cubed
1 medium tomato, finely chopped
1 tablespoon pickled or fresh jalapeño chilli, finely chopped
½ bunch fresh coriander, chopped
½ lime

Method

1. In a large saucepan, combine the water with the garlic, whole onion and 1 teaspoon salt. Bring to the boil, reduce the heat and simmer for 10 minutes. Add the fish and simmer, uncovered, until just cooked through, about 5 minutes. Transfer the fish to a platter to cool. Break the fish into large pieces, discarding any bones and skin.

2. In a large frying pan, heat the coconut oil. Add the chopped onion and sweet potato and cook over high heat, stirring, until just beginning to brown. Add the tomato, and cook, stirring occasionally, until the mixture resembles a hash. Stir in the chilli.

3. Add the fish and cook until warmed through and all the liquid has been absorbed, about 5 minutes. Season to taste and serve in a bowl scattered with coriander and with a squeeze of lime.

Scrambled Eggs with Spring Onion, Chilli and Spinach

Serves 2

1 teaspoon extra-virgin olive oil
1 small red chilli, finely chopped
4 spring onions, trimmed and thinly sliced
4 organic eggs
sea salt and freshly ground black pepper
30g baby spinach

Method

1. Heat the olive oil in a small frying pan over a medium heat. When hot, add the chilli and spring onion and stir-fry for 2–3 minutes.

2. Meanwhile, in a large bowl beat the eggs with salt and pepper.

3. Add the eggs to the pan and stir, using a fork to break them up until cooked to your liking.

4. Serve on a bed of fresh, green spinach.

*top tip

Eggs are one of my favourite foods. They fill you up a treat so are great for breakfast, plus they contain selenium, amino acids and vitamins and so reliably give a great energy boost.

Clean & Lean Super Omelette

Serves 1

sea salt and freshly ground black pepper
100g organic, skinless chicken breast
2 teaspoons extra-virgin olive oil
2–3 organic eggs
30g organic goat's cheese crumbled, or soft goat's cheese
20g baby spinach
½ avocado, peeled and sliced
1 tablespoon chopped chives

Method

1. Preheat a grill plate or barbecue to high.

2. Season the chicken and cook for about 5 minutes on each side, or until cooked through. Remove from the heat and slice thinly.

3. Heat the oil in a small frying pan. Beat the eggs with salt and pepper in a bowl and tip into the pan, lifting up the edges of the omelette with a spatula to avoid sticking.

4. When the omelette is beginning to set, place the chicken, cheese, spinach and avocado on top and cook for 1 minute further, then remove from the pan and sprinkle the chives on top.

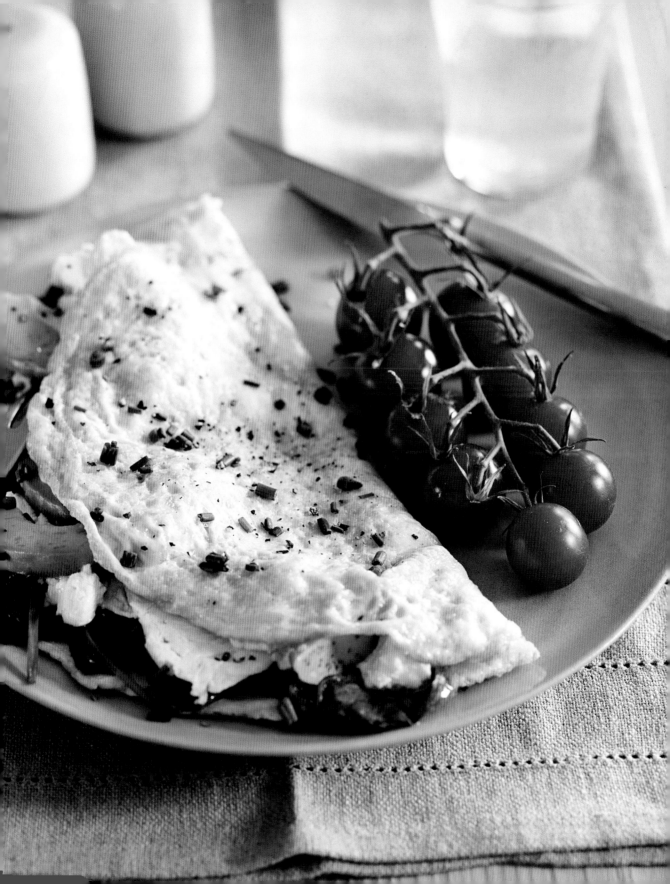

Bodyism Pancakes

Serves 2–4

100g rolled oats
200g fat-free cottage cheese
4 organic eggs
1 teaspoon cinnamon
vegetable or coconut oil
berries, of your choice, to serve

Method

1. Blend the oats, cheese, eggs and cinnamon in a food processor.

2. Heat a little oil in a large frying pan. Pour a ladleful of batter into the pan and cook for 2–3 minutes on each side. Repeat with the remaining mixture.

3. Serve with your favourite berries.

Perfect Porridge with a Mix of Nuts and Seeds

Serves 1

35g rolled oats
2 Brazil nuts, chopped
3 walnuts, chopped
5 almonds, chopped
1 teaspoon pumpkin seeds
½ teaspoon flax seeds
250ml almond or rice milk

Method

1. Soak the oats, nuts and seeds overnight in the almond or rice milk.

2. The next morning, place the porridge mix in a medium saucepan and bring to the boil. Simmer for 5 minutes, stirring regularly.

3. Serve in a bowl with a few extra nuts and seeds sprinkled on top.

Clean & Lean Buckwheat and Banana Pancakes with Pecans

Makes 8/Serves 4

55g wholemeal flour
55g buckwheat flour
275ml milk
1 organic egg
1 banana, mashed
vegetable oil, for frying
manuka honey, for drizzling
60g pecans, chopped

Method

1. In a large bowl, combine the flours and make a well in the centre. Whisk the milk and egg together, then gradually add to the flours and whisk well until you have a smooth batter. Stir in the banana.

2. Heat a little oil in a small frying pan, then pour in a small ladleful of batter and cook for 2–3 minutes each side. Repeat with the remaining mixture.

3. Serve with a drizzle of manuka honey and a scattering of pecans.

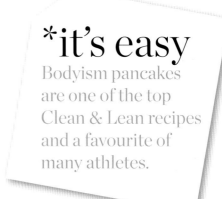

*it's easy
Bodyism pancakes are one of the top Clean & Lean recipes and a favourite of many athletes.

Salmon and Avocado on Rye Toast

Serves 2

2 slices rye bread, toasted
a little butter
100g smoked salmon
1 avocado, halved and sliced
½ lemon
sea salt and freshly ground black pepper

Method

1. Spread the butter on the toast and arrange the salmon and avocado on top.

2. Squeeze some lemon juice over the salmon and season to taste.

Natural Yogurt with Berries and Nuts

Serves 2

100ml organic natural yogurt
60g pecans
100g blueberries
1 teaspoon ground cinnamon
1 teaspoon chia seeds
1 teaspoon ground flaxseed

Method

1. Spoon the yogurt into a bowl and top with the pecans and blueberries.

2. Sprinkle with the cinnamon, chia seeds and flaxseed and serve immediately.

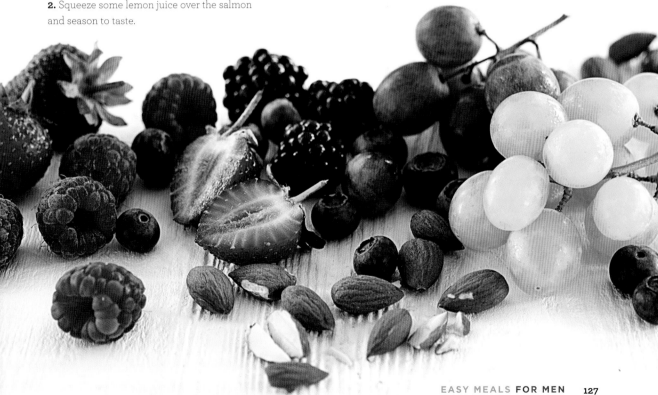

Turkey Loaf

Serves 4

2 tablespoons extra-virgin olive oil
½ medium brown onion, peeled and
   finely chopped
2 cloves garlic, peeled and crushed
450g turkey mince
2 teaspoons fresh thyme leaves
2 medium carrots, grated
1 medium courgette, grated
1 tablespoon pinenuts
1 organic egg, beaten
60ml milk
40g oatmeal
30g Parmesan cheese, finely grated
sea salt and freshly ground black pepper

for the salad
200g rocket leaves
45g dried cranberries
1 small green cucumber, roughly chopped
juice of ½ lemon
sea salt and freshly ground black pepper

Method

1. Heat the oven to 180°C/350°F/gas mark 4.

2. Heat the oil in a small frying pan over medium heat, then cook the onion and garlic until translucent.

3. Line the base of a 28 x 18cm baking tin with greaseproof paper.

4. Mix the remaining meatloaf ingredients together in a large bowl and add the onion and garlic. Season, then transfer the mixture to the baking tin and cook for 30 minutes in the oven, or until cooked through. Finish under the grill for a golden, crispy top.

5. Combine the ingredients for the salad in a medium serving bowl. Slice the loaf and serve with salad.

Clean & Lean Lettuce Wrap

Serves 2

8 raw prawns, peeled
2 teaspoons extra-virgin olive oil
1 clove garlic, peeled and crushed
sea salt and freshly ground black pepper
4 large iceberg lettuce leaves
2 tablespoons guacamole (see recipe
   on page 130)
2 tablespoons tomato salsa (see recipe
   on page 139)
2 tablespoons tinned pinto beans, drained
   and rinsed
1 tablespoon sliced jalapeño chilli,
   finely chopped

Method

1. Toss the prawns in oil and garlic; season to taste. Heat a large frying pan or grill plate over high heat and cook the prawns for about 2 minutes on each side or until cooked through. Remove from the heat.

2. Top each lettuce leaf with 2 garlic prawns, ½ tablespoon guacamole, ½ tablespoon tomato salsa, ½ tablespoon pinto beans and a sprinkling of chilli. Roll them up as for a wrap.

*it's easy
Salmon, spinach, red chilli and Greek yogurt also makes a good filling for a lettuce wrap.

Nutty Super Salad

Serves 1

50g green beans, roughly chopped
50g frozen peas
50g broccoli, roughly chopped
50g carrots, roughly chopped
50g tinned black beans, drained and rinsed
50g almonds, roughly chopped
50g pistachios, roughly chopped
2 tablespoons roughly chopped fresh
    flat-leaf parsley
2 tablespoons roughly chopped fresh
    mint leaves

for the dressing
1½ tablespoons extra-virgin olive oil
1 tablespoon soy sauce
2cm piece of fresh ginger, finely grated
    or chopped

Method
1. Steam, boil or microwave the vegetables
until just cooked.

2. Whisk the dressing ingredients together
in a small bowl.

3. In a large bowl, combine all the ingredients
and drizzle with the dressing.

Clean & Lean Sandwich

Serves 2

2 teaspoons dijon mustard
2 sprouted-grain wraps
100g organic sliced turkey breast
1 avocado, sliced
60g goat's cheese, crumbled

Method
1. Spread 1 teaspoon of mustard over the
centre of each wrap.

2. Top with the turkey, avocado and goat's
cheese, then roll up and enjoy!

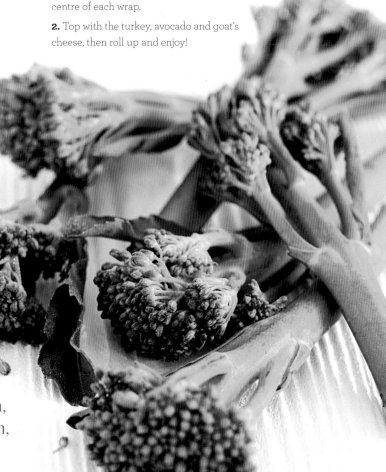

*top tip
If you want to up your protein,
always feel free to add chicken,
a couple of eggs or a portion
of fish.

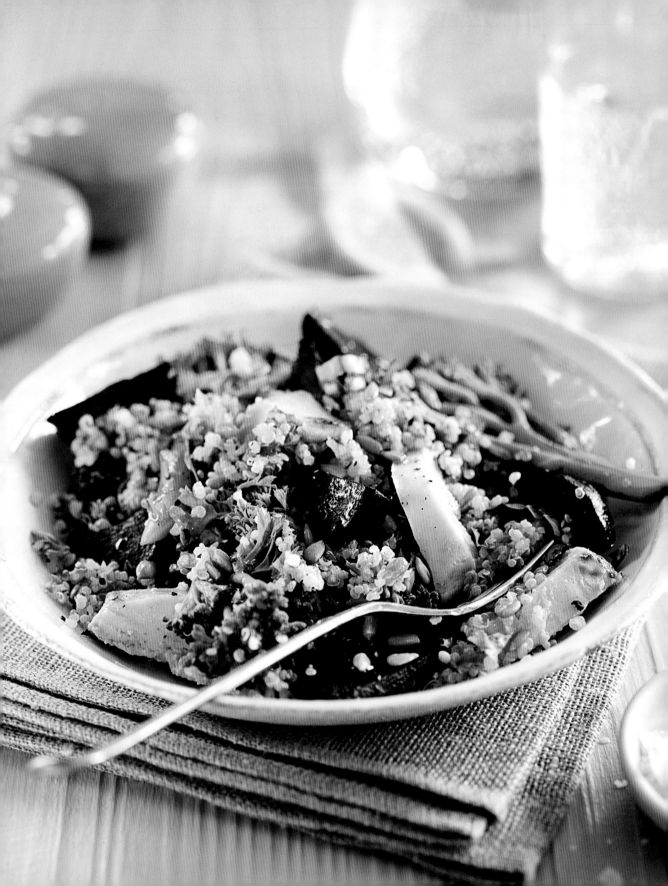

David Gandy's Super Salad

Serves 4

100g Greek yogurt
2 tablespoons dijon mustard
a dash of Tabasco
juice of 1 lemon
sea salt and freshly ground black pepper
4 x 150g skinless organic chicken breasts
3 tablespoons extra-virgin olive oil
4 medium beetroots, trimmed
75g quinoa
1 small broccoli, cut into florets
50g toasted sunflower seeds
½ bunch fresh flat-leaf parsley,
  roughly chopped
½ bunch fresh basil, roughly
  chopped

Method

1. Preheat the oven to 200°C/400°F/gas mark 6.

2. In a large bowl, mix the yogurt, mustard, tabasco and a squeeze of lemon and season to taste. Add the chicken to the bowl and turn to coat.

3. Rub 1 tablespoon of the oil over the beetroot and season to taste. Wrap each in foil and roast for 45 minutes or until tender when pierced with a skewer. Cool, then peel and roughly chop.

4. Transfer the chicken to a non-stick baking tray and bake in the oven for 15–20 minutes.

5. Meanwhile, cook the quinoa according to packet instructions. Steam the broccoli.

6. Mix all the broccoli, beetroots, sunflower seeds, quinoa and herbs in a large bowl. Mix in the remaining 2 tablespoons of the oil and the remaining lemon juice and season to taste.

7. Arrange the quinoa salad in 4 bowls and top each with a sliced chicken breast.

Clean & Lean Superfood Chicken Salad

Serves 4

juice of 1 lime
1 tablespoon manuka honey
1½ tablespoons extra-virgin olive oil
sea salt and freshly ground black pepper
600g organic skinless chicken breasts
1 large butternut squash, peeled and sliced
  into cubes
200g purple sprouting broccoli
150g quinoa, rinsed
1 medium red pepper, trimmed and
  finely chopped
1 avocado, peeled and sliced into cubes
½ bunch fresh mint, leaves roughly
  chopped

for the dressing
60ml extra-virgin olive oil
2 tablespoons balsamic vinegar

Method

1. In a small bowl, combine the lime juice, honey and ½ tablespoon of the oil and season to taste. Add the chicken and coat completely with the marinade. Cover and refrigerate for at least 1 hour.

2. Preheat the oven to 200°C/400°F/gas mark 6.

3. In a bowl, toss the butternut squash with remaining 1 tablespoon oil and season well. Transfer to a large baking tray and roast for 20 minutes.

3. Turn the grill onto medium high. Lift the chicken from the marinade and add to the baking tray with the squash. Place under the grill and cook for 8–10 minutes, turning once, until cooked through. Set aside to cool.

4. Meanwhile, steam the broccoli and cook the quinoa according to packet instructions.

5. Place the pepper and avocado in a large bowl and add the quinoa and cooled butternut squash. Whisk together the ingredients for the dressing and season. Then pour over the salad and toss to coat.

6. To serve, arrange the salad on a plate, and top with the broccoli and a few slices of grilled chicken. Scatter with mint.

Homemade Hummus

200g tinned chickpeas, rinsed and drained
2 tablespoons lemon juice (or more)
2 cloves garlic, peeled and crushed
1 teaspoon ground cumin
100ml tahini (sesame seed paste) optional
60ml water
sea salt
2 tablespoons extra-virgin olive oil
½ teaspoon paprika

Method

1. Reserve a few chickpeas for serving. In a food processor, combine the remaining chickpeas, lemon juice, garlic, cumin, tahini (if using) and water and blend to a creamy purée. Season to taste with extra juice, garlic, cumin or salt if required.

2. Pour into a serving bowl, drizzle with oil and scatter with the reserved chickpeas. Sprinkle with paprika and serve with warm pitta bread.

Hummus and mint salad

Serves 1

40g wild rocket leaves
1 small red pepper, deseeded and sliced
½ bunch fresh mint, leaves roughly torn
sea salt and freshly ground black pepper
2 tablespoons homemade hummus
   (see left)
a little organic butter
2 slices rye bread or wholegrain flatbreads,
   toasted

Method

1. Put the rocket on a plate, sprinkle the pepper and the mint on top and season to taste. Spoon the hummus on top.

2. Butter the bread and serve with the salad.

Guacamole

Serves 4

1 medium tomato, roughly chopped
juice of 1 lime
½ small red onion, peeled and
   roughly chopped
1 large green chilli, finely chopped
1 small bunch coriander, leaves roughly
   chopped
sea salt, to taste
2 ripe avocados, halved and peeled

Method

Place all the ingredients except the avocado in a blender and whizz for 20 seconds or until finely chopped. Add the avocado and whizz for 20 more seconds or until the desired consistency is reached.

*it's easy
Homemade hummus is great because you know exactly what is in it, and it tastes much better too.

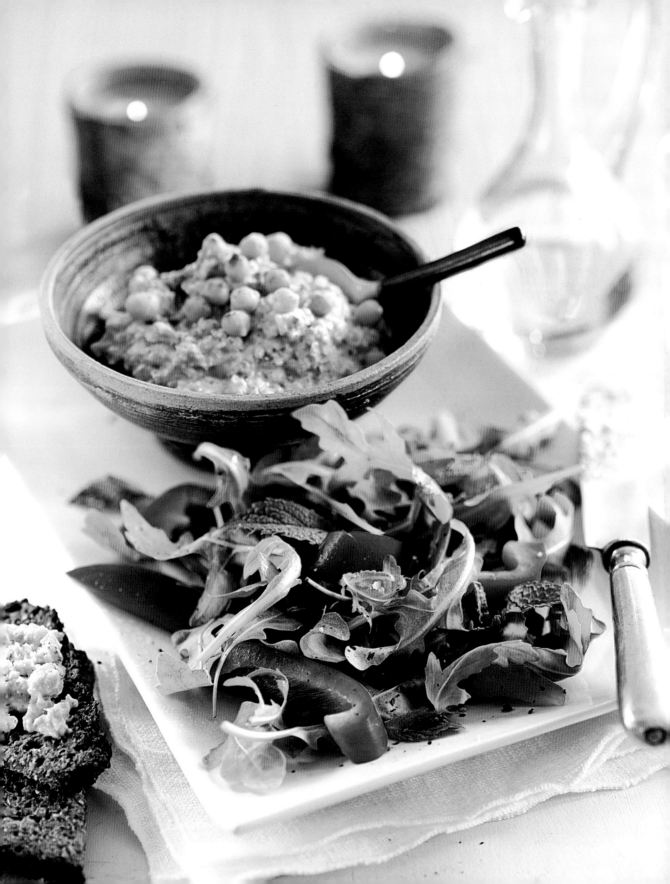

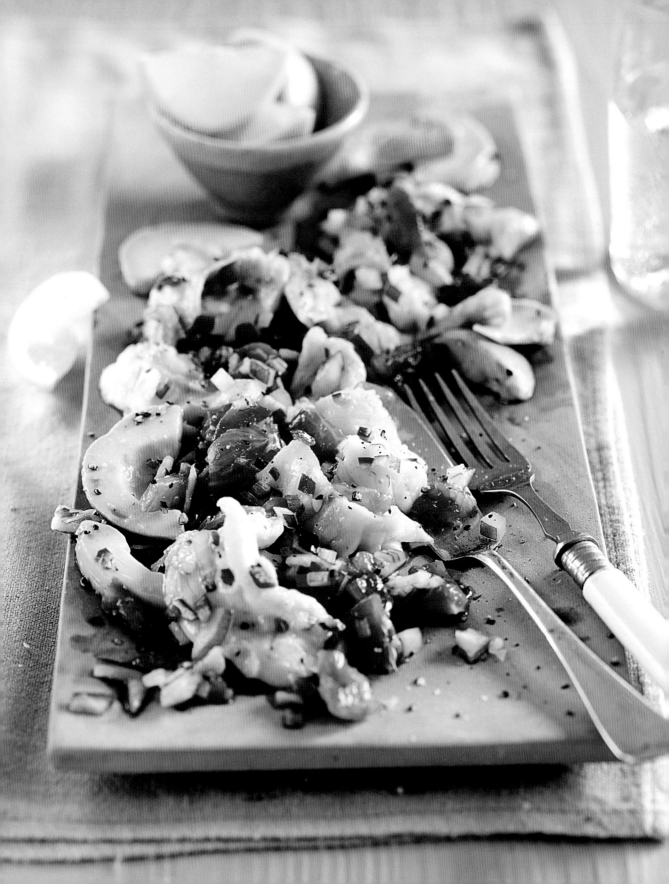

Ceviche

Serves 4

400g sashimi-grade sea bass fillet, skin
   removed, thinly sliced
juice of 2 limes
juice of 1½ lemons
½ medium red onion, peeled and chopped
4 medium ripe tomatoes, peeled and
   deseeded
1 small red chilli, finely chopped
sea salt and freshly ground black pepper
1 avocado, sliced

Method

1. In a bowl, mix all the ingredients except the
avocado and leave to marinate in the fridge
for about 15 minutes or up to 1 hour.

2. Drain the juice and discard. Serve with
freshly sliced avocado and an extra squeeze
of lemon.

Beetroot, Walnut, Spinach and Goat's Cheese Salad

Serves 4

4 medium fresh beetroot, trimmed and
   peeled
4 cloves garlic, peeled
2 tablespoons aged balsamic vinegar
2 tablespoons extra-virgin olive oil
200g baby spinach leaves or salad greens
200g goat's cheese, crumbled
100g walnuts, chopped
1 tablespoon fresh tarragon leaves

Method

1. Preheat the oven to 200°C/400°F/gas
mark 6.

2. Wrap each beetroot together with a
garlic clove in foil and roast in the oven for
approximately 45 minutes or until tender
when pierced with a skewer. Leave to cool,
then cut into small wedges.

3. Meanwhile, whisk together the vinegar and
oil. Arrange the spinach on a plate and place
the beetroot on top. Drizzle with the dressing
and then scatter with the goat's cheese,
walnuts and tarragon.

*top tip
There are unusually high
nitrate levels in beetroot
and studies indicate it can
reduce blood pressure
as effectively as many
clinical drugs.

Grilled Chicken, Brown Rice and Black Beans

Serves 2

2 x 150g organic skinless chicken breasts
1 tablespoon extra-virgin olive oil
1 small brown onion, peeled and diced
2 cloves garlic, peeled and crushed
2 large ripe tomatoes, peeled and
   finely chopped
1 tablespoon finely chopped pimento peppers
300g tinned black beans, drained and rinsed
115g brown rice
200ml water
2 tablespoons fresh coriander leaves,
   roughly chopped
2 tablespoons fresh flat-leaf parsley,
   roughly chopped
sea salt
1 pinch cayenne pepper
½ lime, quartered, to serve

for the marinade
1 tablespoon balsamic vinegar
1 tablespoon honey
juice of 1 lime
1 pinch cayenne pepper

Method

1. Mix the marinade ingredients in a bowl and add the chicken, turning to coat. Cover and refrigerate for at least 1 hour.

2. Preheat the grill to high. Lift the chicken from the marinade and place on a baking tray. Grill for 8 minutes on each side, or until cooked through. Remove from the heat and rest for 5 minutes before slicing.

3. Meanwhile, heat the oil in a large saucepan over a medium heat. Add the onion and cook, stirring occasionally, until translucent. Add the garlic, tomatoes and pimentos. Stir in the beans, rice, water, herbs, salt to taste and cayenne pepper. Bring to the boil, reduce the heat and simmer until all the water is absorbed, about 12 minutes.

4. Check the rice is thoroughly cooked. Divide between plates and serve with the chicken, an extra sprinkle of coriander and a lime wedge on the side.

Greek Lamb Salad

Serves 2

½ lemon, zest and juice
2 stalks rosemary, leaves finely chopped
1 clove garlic, peeled and crushed
1 tablespoon extra-virgin olive oil
1 x 300g lamb steak
sea salt
1 little gem lettuce, leaves torn
200g baby spinach leaves
1 large ripe tomato, roughly chopped
1 small green cucumber, roughly chopped
80g black olives, pitted
100g feta cheese, crumbled

for the dressing:
45ml extra-virgin olive oil
45ml lemon juice
1 clove garlic, peeled and crushed

Method

1. In a bowl, mix the zest, juice, rosemary, garlic and oil. Add the lamb and turn to coat. Refrigerate for an hour or so.

2. Preheat a grill or grill pan. Season the lamb with salt and grill over a high heat for 4 minutes on each side or until cooked to your liking. Remove from the heat and rest for 5 minutes.

3. Meanwhile, in a small bowl, whisk the dressing ingredients together. In a medium serving bowl, mix the lettuce, spinach, tomato, cucumber, olives and cheese and toss with the dressing.

4. Slice the lamb across the grain and serve with the salad.

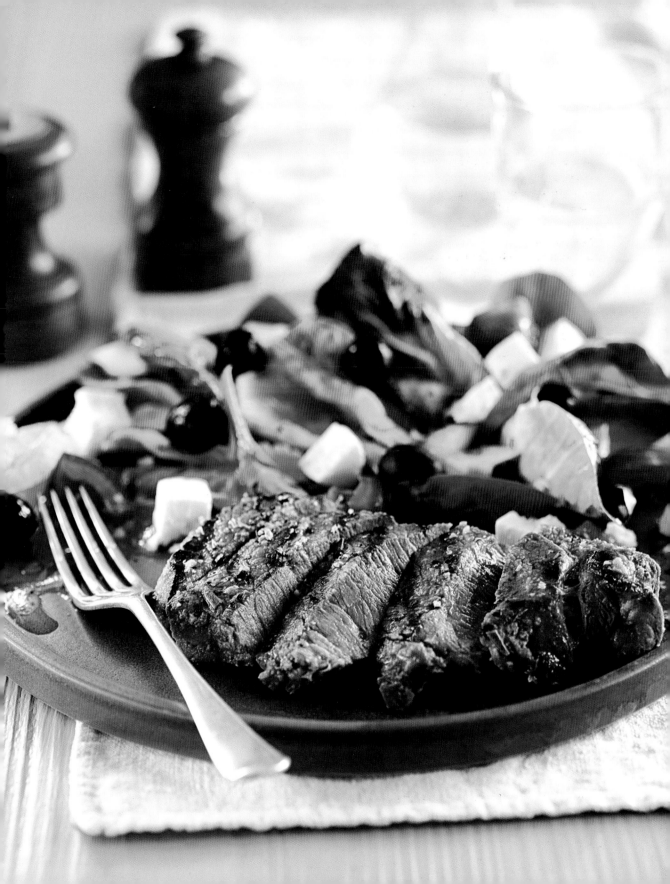

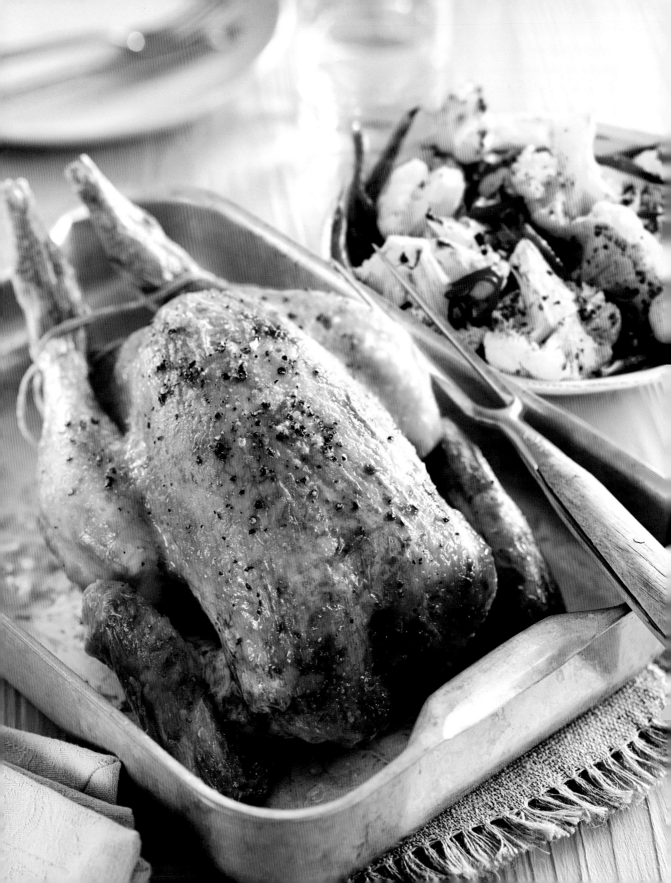

Roast Organic Chicken and Roast Cauliflower with Garlic and Chilli

Serves 4

1.2kg whole organic chicken
1 lemon, zested, then cut in half
2 cloves garlic, peeled and halved
2 tablespoons extra-virgin olive oil
sea salt and freshly ground black pepper
400g cauliflower florets
1 clove garlic, peeled and crushed
2 small red chillies, finely sliced
¼ teaspoon turmeric

Method

1. Preheat the oven to 220°C/425°F/gas mark 7.

2. Clean the chicken inside and out with cool running water. Pat dry inside and out with absorbent kitchen paper. Stuff the chicken with the lemon and the halved garlic cloves. Rub 1 tablespoon of the oil into the skin and season well all over.

3. Place on a roasting rack breast-side down. Roast the chicken for 20 minutes, then reduce the oven temperature to 180°C/350°F/gas mark 4 and roast for a further hour, or until cooked through.

4. Once the chicken has been roasting for an hour, combine the cauliflower in a bowl with the crushed garlic, chilli, turmeric and remaining oil and season to taste. Spread out in an ovenproof dish in a single layer.

5. Roast, uncovered, for 20 minutes or until the floret tops are lightly browned. Remove from the oven and serve immediately with the roast chicken.

*top tip

Don't be limited by the proteins we include here. If you can find game like venison or rabbit or elk or buffalo or caribou...

Warm Quinoa Salad with Chicken and Eggs

Serves 1

50g quinoa, rinsed
3 broccoli florets
2 organic eggs
1 cooked chicken breast, pulled apart
  (or leftover roast chicken)
sea salt and freshly ground black pepper

Method

1. Cook the quinoa according to packet instructions. Steam the broccoli.

2. Bring a pan of water to the boil and poach or soft-boil the eggs.

3. Add the eggs to the warm bowl of quinoa, then add the chicken and stir to break up the egg yolk. Season to taste and serve with the steamed broccoli.

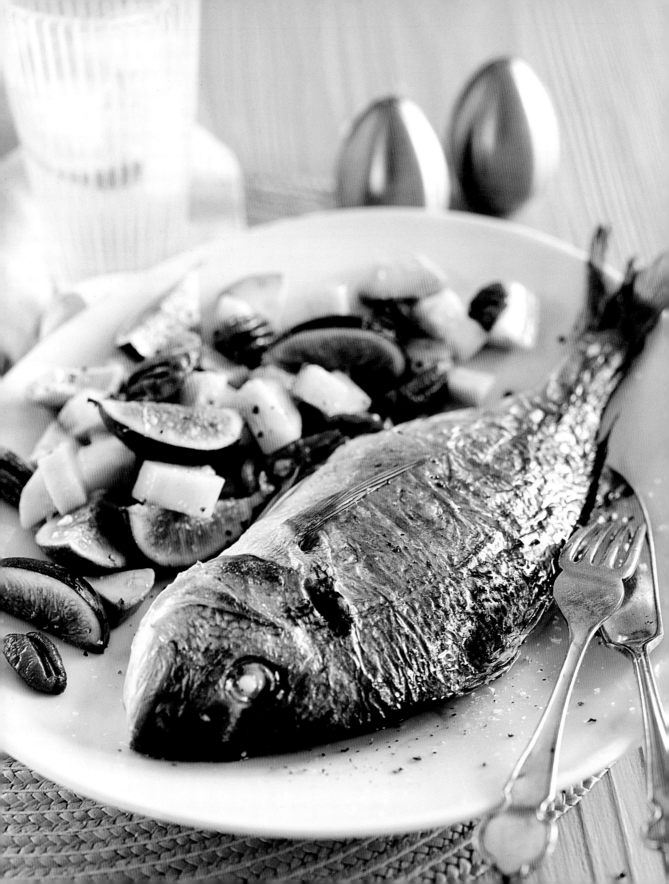

Sea Bass with Tomato Salsa

Serves 4

sea salt and freshly ground black pepper
1 tablespoon extra-virgin olive oil
4 x 200g sea bass fillets
2 tablespoons fresh oregano, chopped

for the tomato salsa
500g ripe tomatoes, peeled, deseeded and
 finely chopped
2 tablespoons extra-virgin olive oil
1 medium shallot or small red onion, peeled
 and finely chopped
juice of ¼ lemon
sea salt and freshly ground black pepper
2 tablespoons fresh oregano, chopped

Method

1. Preheat the oven to 180°C/350°F/gas mark 4.

2. Make the salsa by tossing all the ingredients together in a large bowl.

3. Season and drizzle a little oil over the sea bass and bake in the oven for 15–20 minutes or until cooked through.

4. Serve the fish with the salsa, sprinkle the oregano on top and eat with a pile of your favourite vegetables.

Crispy Baked Sea Bream with a Pecan, Cucumber, Fig and Avocado Salad

Serves 2

4 tablespoons extra-virgin olive oil
2 x 400g whole sea bream, scaled and
 gutted
sea salt and freshly ground black pepper
1 Lebanese or English cucumber, peeled
 and roughly chopped
80g pecan halves
1 avocado, chopped into cubes
4 fresh figs, cut into quarters
1 small bunch mint, roughly chopped
juice of ½ lemon

Method

1. Preheat the oven to 220°C/425°F/gas mark 7.

2. Pour 1 tablespoon of the oil into a large, ovenproof dish. Lay the fish in the dish and cut a slash into each side of the fish about 1cm deep. Rub 1 tablespoon oil into the skin, season to taste and roast for 25 minutes.

3. Mix the remaining ingredients together in a bowl with the rest of the oil. Season to taste and serve each fish with the salad on the side.

*it's easy
Fishtofork.com is a great resource for information on the most sustainable fish to eat.

JAMES' FAVOURITE STEAK

Being Australian, I love a good steak. In fact, I'd say it was in the top five of my favourite foods ever. However, I limit myself to no more than one a week and I always eat the best-quality steak I can get. It's far better to have an expensive steak once every so often than it is to eat loads of cheap, non-organic supermarket steak and mince several times a week.

I've eaten steaks all over the world and my favourite is a rib eye, at least 2 inches high, seared until it looks perfect and roasted with rosemary and garlic until medium rare. I also like it sprinkled with Himalayan sea salt, sliced on a big wooden chopping board and served with sweet potato mash and sautéed spinach.

Why I like it...

Steak is a fantastic source of iron which boosts your energy levels. And although iron is fairly hard for the body to absorb, the following vitamins help your body absorb it more efficiently, so try to serve these alongside your steak:
✳ Vitamin C: found in citrus fruits, strawberries, kiwi fruits, Brussels sprouts, cauliflower, kale (a dark green leafy vegetable) and peppers
✳ Vitamin A: found in sweet potatoes, carrots, broccoli, peas and lemons

Note: a few things can actually inhibit the absorption of iron, including the tannin found in tea and the calcium in milk, so avoid these when eating steak.

Grilled Rib-Eye Steak with Sweet Potato Mash and Chilli Broccoli

Serves 4

2 small sweet potatoes, peeled and roughly chopped
2 tablespoons organic Greek yogurt
3 tablespoons pomegranate seeds
sea salt and freshly ground black pepper
4 x 200g grass-fed rib-eye steaks
35ml sesame oil
1 large broccoli, broken into florets
1 small red chilli, finely chopped

Method

1. Place the sweet potato in a medium saucepan and just cover with water. Bring to the boil and cook, uncovered, for about 8 minutes or until very soft. Drain and transfer to a large bowl and mash with the yogurt. Stir in the pomegranate seeds and season to taste.

2. Meanwhile, heat a grill pan until very hot. Rub the steaks with 2 tablespoons of the sesame oil and season. Cook for about 3 minutes on each side for medium rare. Rest for 5–10 minutes.

3. Steam the broccoli, then transfer to a bowl. Drizzle with the remaining sesame oil and sprinkle with the chilli.

4. Serve the steak with the mash and broccoli on the side.

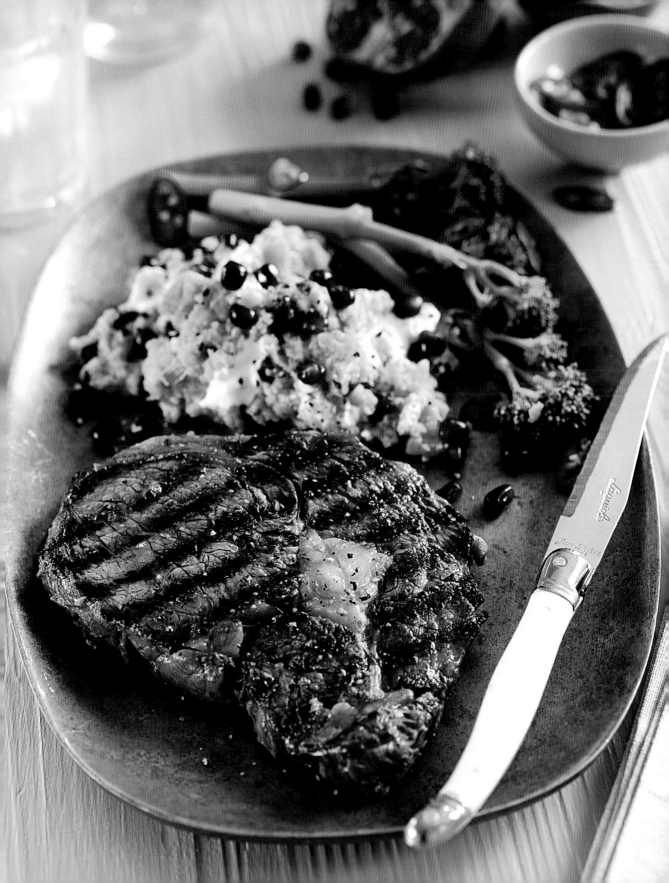

Braised Beef Short Ribs with Roasted Vegetables

Serves 4

3 tablespoons macadamia nut oil (or olive oil)
6 x 150g beef short ribs with bones
sea salt and freshly ground black pepper
1 large brown onion, peeled and finely chopped
3 cloves garlic, peeled and sliced
750ml red wine
700ml chicken stock
1 small butternut squash, peeled and cubed
1 small sweet potato, peeled and cubed
2 medium parsnips, peeled and sliced lengthways
3 medium carrots, peeled and sliced lengthways
1 bunch fresh flat-leaf parsley, roughly chopped

Method

1. Heat 2 tablespoons of the oil in a large frying pan over a high heat. Season the ribs with salt and pepper and add them to the pan. Cook over a moderate heat, turning once, until brown, about 10 minutes. Transfer the ribs to a large ovenproof casserole.

2. Add the onion and garlic to the frying pan and sauté until lightly browned. Add the wine and bring to the boil. Pour the pan contents over the ribs and leave to cool. Cover and refrigerate overnight, turning the ribs once.

3. Preheat the oven to 180°C/350°F/gas mark 4.

4. Add the stock to the ribs, place over a moderate heat and bring to the boil. Cover, transfer to the oven and cook for 1½ hours. Uncover and braise for 45 minutes longer, turning the ribs once or twice, until the sauce is reduced by about half and the meat is very tender.

5. Meanwhile, arrange the vegetables in a single layer in a large roasting pan, season and toss in 1 tablespoon of oil. Add the vegetables to the oven 30 minutes before the end of the cooking time for the ribs; cook for about 30 minutes. Remove from the oven and keep warm.

6. Preheat the grill. Transfer the meat to a clean baking dish, discarding the bones as they fall off. Strain the sauce into a heatproof bowl and then pour over the meat.

7. Place the meat under the grill and cook for about 10 minutes, turning once or twice, until glazed and sizzling.

8. Serve with the roasted root vegetables and a sprinkling of parsley.

JAMES' FAVOURITE DINNER

Thai Chicken Curry

Serves 2

100g brown rice
160ml water
1 tablespoon vegetable oil
5 spring onions, trimmed and sliced
1 clove garlic, peeled and crushed
2½cm piece fresh ginger, peeled and thinly sliced
2 small green chillies, thinly sliced
1 stalk lemongrass, white part finely chopped
4 x 200g organic skinless chicken thigh fillets, roughly chopped
200ml coconut milk
juice of 1 lime
2 tablespoons fresh coriander leaves

Method

1. Rinse the rice and combine with the water in a medium saucepan over a high heat. Bring to boil, reduce the heat and simmer, covered, for 30 minutes or until the water has been absorbed. Keep the lid on and rest for up to 10 minutes.

2. While the rice is resting, heat the oil in a large frying pan over a high heat. Add the onions, garlic, ginger, chilli and lemongrass and cook, stirring until just brown. Add the chicken and cook until brown.

3. Add the coconut milk and water and simmer for 5 minutes.

4. Remove from the heat, stir in the lime juice and top with the coriander. Serve with the rice.

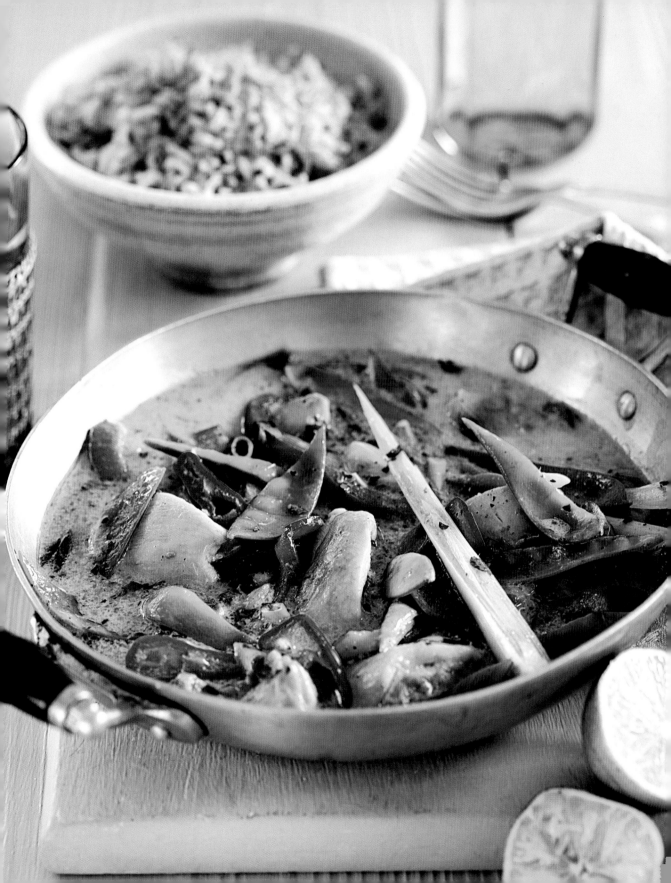

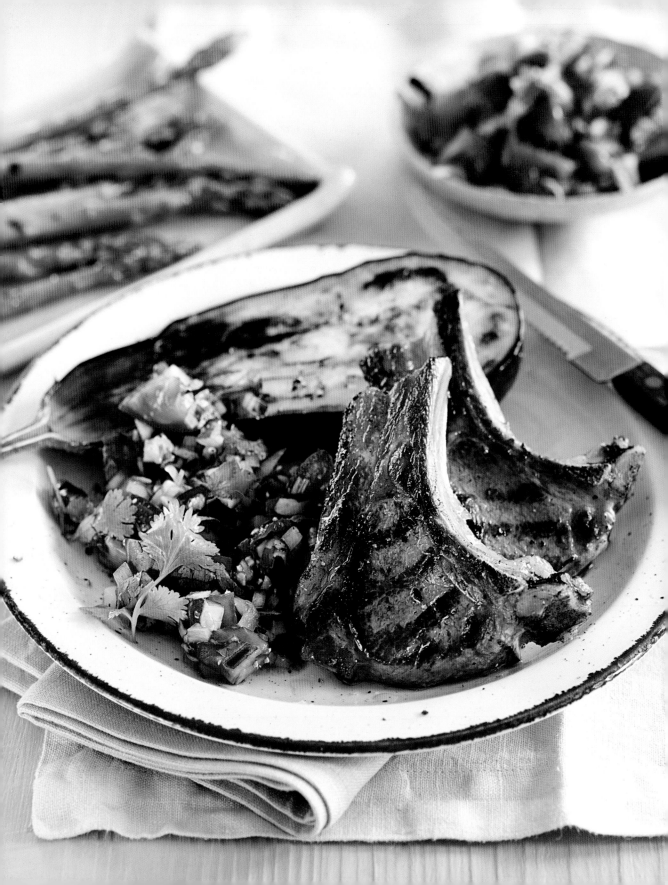

Lamb Cutlets with Baked Aubergine, Tomato Salsa and Grilled Asparagus

Serves 4

4 tablespoons extra-virgin olive oil
2 large aubergines, halved
sea salt and freshly ground black pepper
2 bunches of asparagus
8 x 60g lamb cutlets
2 large, ripe tomatoes, diced
½ red onion, peeled and diced
½ bunch fresh coriander, leaves chopped
juice of 2 limes

Method

1. Heat 2 tablespoons of the oil in a large frying pan. Sauté the aubergine, with a pinch of salt, until tender. Allow to cool a little.

2. Heat a grill pan until very hot. Toss the asparagus in 1 tablespoon of the oil and cook, turning occasionally, until nicely marked and browned on all sides. Transfer to a plate.

3. Drizzle the lamb with the remaining 1 tablespoon of the oil and season to taste. Cook on the grill pan for about 3 minutes on each side or until cooked.

4. In a large bowl, mix together the tomatoes, onion, coriander and lime juice.

5. Serve the lamb cutlets with the salsa, aubergine and asparagus on the side.

*top tip

These are delicious cooked over a hot barbecue but a preheated griddle pan works well too.

Spicy Quinoa Muscle Salad

Serves 1

180g quinoa
2 teaspoons coconut oil
1 medium onion, peeled and chopped
1 fresh green chilli, chopped
2 garlic cloves, peeled and chopped
230ml chicken or vegetable stock
1 salmon fillet (or another protein – sea bass, chicken thighs, turkey thighs)
sea salt and freshly ground black pepper
a handful of fresh coriander, freshly chopped
10 walnuts, halved
5 spring onions, trimmed and chopped
2 tablespoons lime juice
¼ teaspoon salt

Method

1. Preheat the grill to high.

2. Toast the quinoa in a large dry pan over medium heat, stirring frequently until it begins to colour (3–5 minutes).

3. Heat the oil in a large saucepan over medium heat. Add the onion and cook until translucent, then add the chilli and garlic. Add the quinoa and stock, bring to the boil, then reduce to a gentle simmer. Cover and cook until the quinoa is tender and most of the liquid has been absorbed, 20–25 minutes.

4. Meanwhile, season the salmon with salt and pepper, place on a baking tray and grill until cooked all the way through.

5. Add the coriander, walnuts, spring onions, lime juice and salt to the quinoa, mix gently and fluff with a fork.

6. Serve the salmon on top of the quinoa with a squeeze of lime.

*top tip

Manuka honey is rich in antibacterial and antifungal properties and has many health benefits. If you can't beat that sweet craving, drizzle a teaspoon over a bowl of organic Greek yogurt or this quinoa pudding.

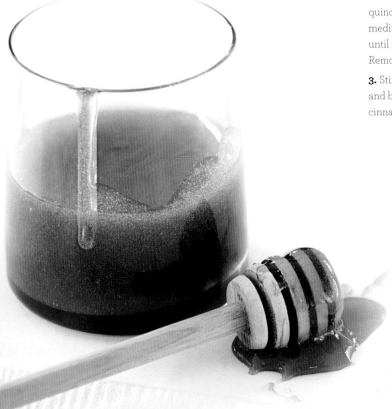

Quinoa Pudding

Serves 2

100g quinoa

110ml rice or almond milk

1 scoop Vanilla Protein Excellence (optional, cleanandlean.com)

50g berries (of your choice)

1 teaspoon cinnamon

35g toasted almonds

Method

1. Rinse and drain the quinoa, then cook according to the packet instructions.

2. Combine the rice or almond milk and quinoa in a saucepan and cook over a medium heat for about 5–10 minutes, stirring until the mixture becomes thick and creamy. Remove from the heat.

3. Stir in the Vanilla Protein Excellence and berries and serve warm, sprinkled with cinnamon and toasted almonds.

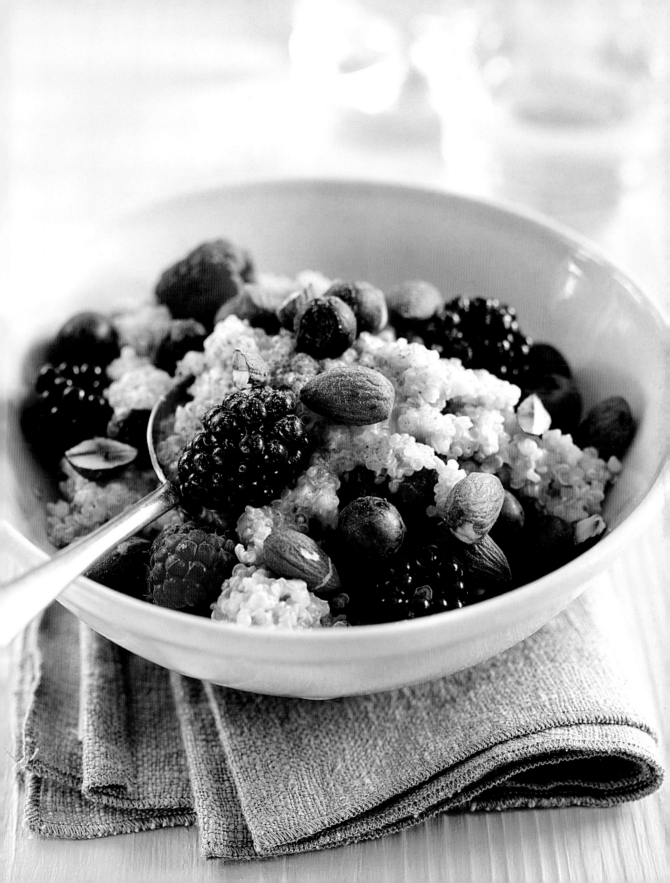

Frozen Yogurt

Serves 4

200g natural yogurt
100g blueberries
100g strawberries
ice cubes
cinnamon

Method

1. Place all the ingredients in a blender and blend to a smooth purée.

2. Pour the mixture into a loaf tin or container, cover with a lid or a tight layer of cling film and freeze overnight, until solid.

3. Remove from the freezer about 10–15 minutes before serving. It can be frozen for up to a month.

*top tip

Always try to find organic, probiotic forms of natural yogurt. They are the best for you.

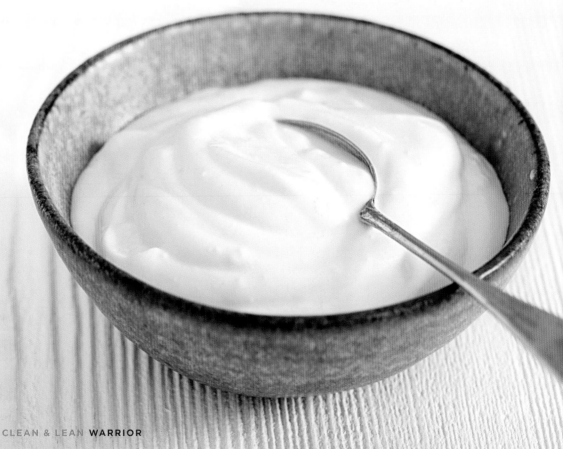

Coconut Macaroons

170g desiccated coconut
2 egg whites
50g pecans
50g sunflower seeds
25g dried apricots

Method

1. Preheat the oven to 180°C/350°F/gas mark 3.

2. Blitz all the ingredients together in a food processor.

3. Roll the mixture into golf-ball sized balls and place, well-spaced, on a baking tray lined with greaseproof paper. Bake for about 15 minutes or until brown. Cool for 5 minutes before transferring to a cake rack to finish cooling.

Raspberry Chocolate Heaven
Serves 1

2 tablespoons ricotta
60g raspberries
1 tablespoon toasted slivered almonds
a sprinkle of cocoa

Method

Spoon the ricotta in to a bowl and top with the rest of the ingredients.

Frozen Yogalato
Serves 4

500g natural yogurt
50g toasted almonds, chopped
50g pecans, chopped
50g raspberries, chopped
50g blueberries, chopped
50g desiccated coconut

Method

1. Mix all the ingredients in a large bowl.

2. Pour the mixture into a loaf tin or container, cover with a lid or a tight layer of cling film and freeze overnight, until solid.

3. Remove from the freezer about 10–15 minutes before you want to serve and enjoy like ice cream.

*top tip

For a frozen yogalato, you can mix your favourite Clean & Lean ingredients as you please.

5 SMOOTHIES THAT WILL MAKE YOU STRONGER

all recipes serve 1

Green Smoothie

400g fresh spinach, trimmed and chopped
1 stick celery
¼ cucumber
2½cm piece fresh ginger
juice of ¼ lemon
3 florets cooked broccoli

Method
Blitz all the ingredients together in a blender.

Warrior Protein Shake

1 scoop Protein Excellence
230ml almond milk
1 teaspoon peanut butter
1 banana
ice cubes

Method
Blitz all the ingredients together in a blender.

Oil-Your-Engine Shake

250ml almond milk
4 ice cubes
1 scoop Protein Excellence
1 teaspoon almond butter
1 tablespoon flax seeds
1 tablespoon chia seeds

Method
Blitz all the ingredients together in a blender.

Blue Nut Shake

250ml milk
2 tablespoons oats
50g blueberries
25g walnuts
25g brazil nuts
½ teaspoon ground cinnamon

Method
Blitz all the ingredients together in a blender.

Super Green Breakfast Smoothie

250ml rice milk
1 scoop Vanilla Protein Excellence
1 teaspoon Ultimate Clean
1 teaspoon Beauty Food
½ teaspoon ground cinnamon
25g walnuts
30g baby spinach leaves
5 mint leaves

Method
Blend all the ingredients together in a blender.

*top tip
All supplements are available online at bodyism.com and cleanandlean.com

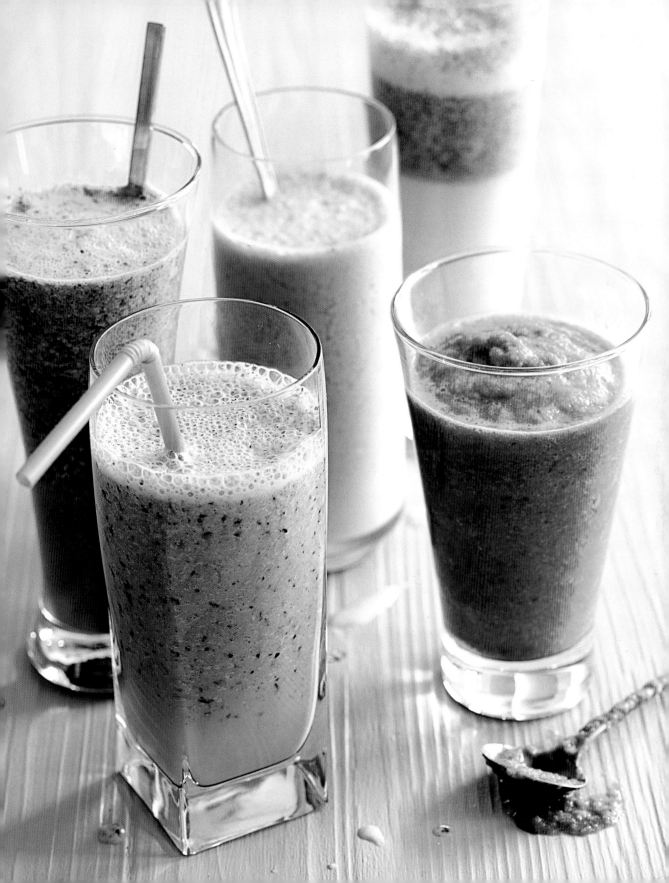

James Duigan

STAY STRONG FOR LIFE

So you've got this far – well done! If you've followed my 14-day Warrior Plan you should be feeling pretty amazing right now. And if you're about to start it, having read the rest of this book, I imagine you're feeling fired up and ready to change your life. Going forwards, I don't expect you to follow every single Clean & Lean rule. You might still want a beer after work or to eat a ready meal when you come home late. And that's fine. But if you take everything I've said in this book, process it and try to live by it as much as you realistically can, you're taking a huge step in the right direction.

Here's a quick at-a-glance reminder of my Clean & Lean rules:

✳ Choose Clean & Lean foods that look like food – not like they were made in a factory.

✳ Eat protein, fat and some vegetables at every meal.

✳ Chew your food properly and don't eat when you're stressed.

✳ Eat brightly coloured, thin-skinned fruit.

✳ Reduce your coffee intake. Stick to one or two cups a day.

✳ Eat good fat – it will boost your energy levels, improve your concentration and give you a 6-pack.

✳ Avoid sugar. It'll make you fat and weak.

✳ Don't drink too much beer – it will make your body look like a woman's!

✳ Channel your rage and work off your stress – get outside and move around a lot. It's the only way you'll feel better.

✳ Do something you enjoy every week. Every day, if possible.

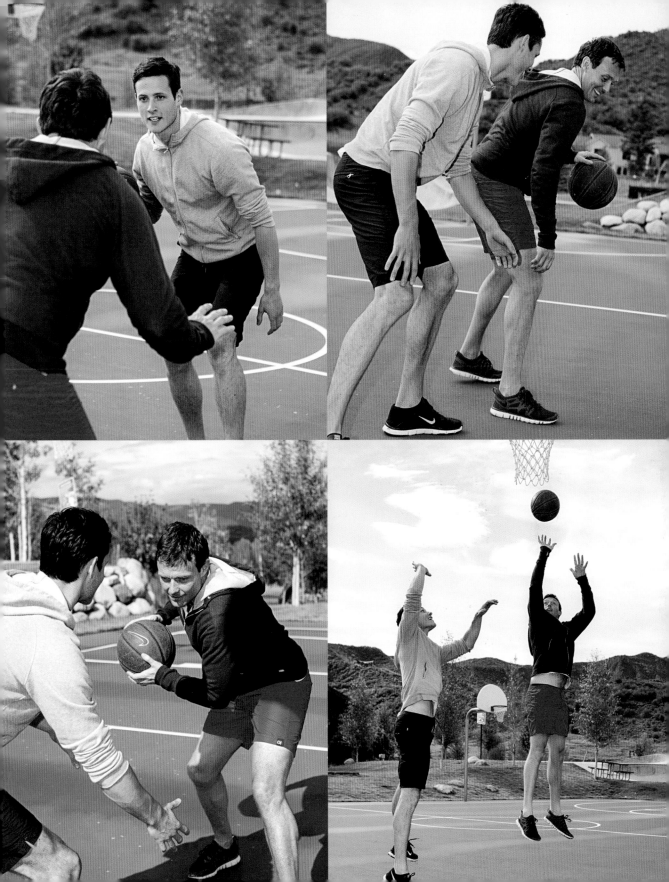

INDEX

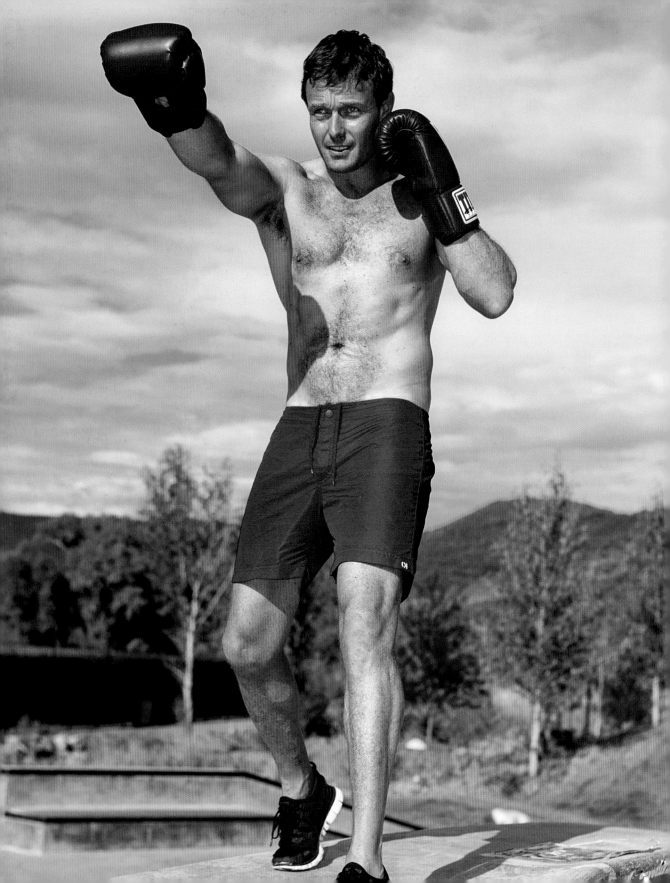

ACKNOWLEDGEMENTS

Thank you to my beautiful wife, Chrissy, for everything. For carrying our little girl in your tummy and for being my best friend and picking me up from the floor when I thought it was all too much. You truly are the most wonderful person in the world. Our little girl, you're not here yet, but we love you so much. My Dad, Kevin Duigan, my hero, they gave you no chance, but we knew better. You faced death with gentle words and an open heart. Your courage and compassion has guided me every day of my life and made me the man I am today. I promise you I'll never let you down. My beautiful mum for raising me to be strong and healthy. My sister for being a brilliant, beautiful soul. The whole family for looking after Dad; and Auntie Angela and Chris for scaring the doctors. Friends Chantal and Luke, Anthony and Tania, Margot and George, Lisa and Faleh, Beth and David, Daisy and Susie and Lisa and Corey, who stood by us when all seemed lost, you were all there when we needed you. Ivan and Marina, your friendship and wisdom gave us strength to get through when we thought we couldn't. Wonderful Tatiana and our friend Joe Dowdell. Brilliant, talented Maria, again! The wonderful Stephanie Haynes, thank you for making a dream come true. Lee and Nat, shoulder to shoulder you stood with us against all odds, you were there every moment and made it all happen while I was broken with sadness. Thank you for being the truest of friends. Nat, you're amazing. Lee, little brother, it's only getting better. The Bodyism team, for officially being the best in the world! Tom and Adam, the two most eligible bachelors in town, we love you too much. Thanks for being there always. Patrice for believing in us, we love you. Hani, you saved us and asked nothing in return. Thank you for being so kind. The people who kicked us when we were down, we forgive you. Thank you for making us stronger and kinder. Elle, for teaching me that a true friend will be there in your time of need without thinking of themselves. Vincent and Sylvain, what a team we are! Tom P, for being so handsome and for being a wonderful soul. My mate Mike, always. Andrew and Kahrina for your passion and patience. Ben Duigan, for everything. Rosie, for being our family, for being generous and kind and brave and brilliant. Holly for being such a wonderful selfless angel. Frank Atkinson, quite literally our hero. The Clean & Lean community for being so inspiring and supportive. Hugh, for being better and kinder than anyone will probably ever know. We love you. Justin Alexander, for being the strongest shoulder to cry on. Finally God, for hearing my prayers. It will all be ok in the end, and if it's not ok, it's not the end . .

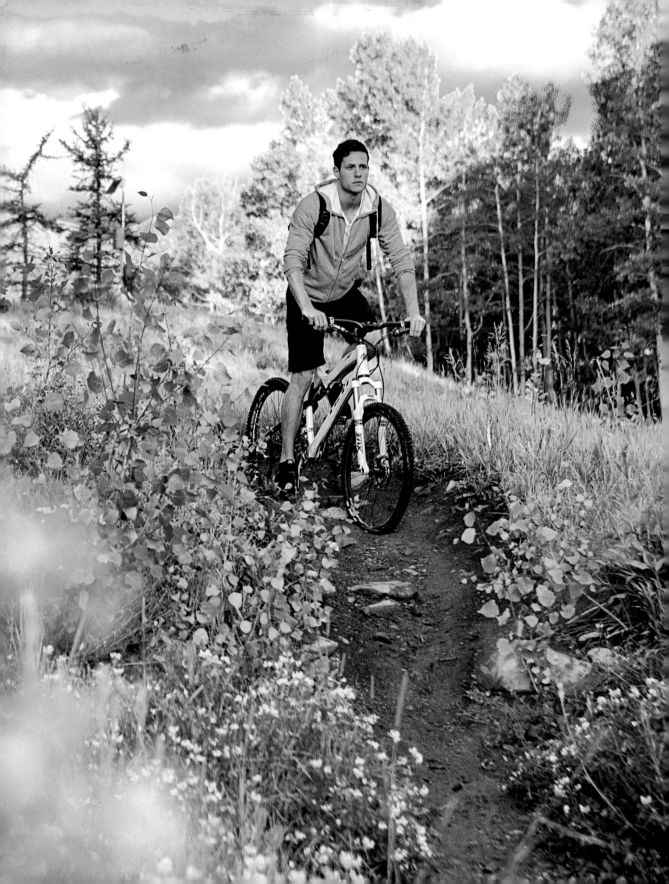